PRAISE FOR THE
ALKALINE APPROACH

"By simply eating a more alkaline diet—veggies, greens, fresh organic green juices and smoothies, sprouts, wheatgrass juice, certain grains, and other fabulous plant foods—you will explode with vibrant energy and well-being." – Kris Carr, author of *Crazy Sexy Diet*

"I have had countless numbers of patients with painful osteoarthritis on many different medications for arthritis. Many have been pain free within a couple of months after adjusting their urine pH to 7.0 to 7.5 by consuming adequate amounts of alkaline water and alkaline foods." – Dr. Colbert, author of *7 Pillars of Health*

"[The Alkaline Cure] is a small, simple set of lifestyle choices, which compound to produce a massive difference when you keep doing them." – Andrew Bridgewater, UK Chartered Psychologist

"Victoria [Beckham] is on the alkaline diet and she swears by it for healthy eating and weight loss ... I feel amazing! ... I thought I knew what I was doing nutrition wise but I'm amazed what a difference alkalizing makes." – Melanie Chisholm (Sporty Spice), in *Hello* magazine

"As long as we do not increase our body's alkalinity, we will never solve the cancer riddle ... It is the excess acid in our body that cultivates cancer..." – Sang Whang, author of *The Cancer Riddle*

"[Mark Ruffalo] switched to a largely plant-based alkaline diet after working with me during The Avengers. He lost weight and told me, 'I feel so great I never want to go back.'" – Kimberly Snyder, nutritionist, *Vogue* magazine

PRAISE FOR THE F.X. MAYR & MORE HEALTH CENTER

"Fellow guests included a Seventies rock star, a manager of a premier league football club, a lady peer, a CEO and a literary agent … Mayr had turned around the way I think about myself and my health … Oh, and I lost sixteen pounds in twelve days." – Robin Derrick, *Vogue* magazine

"Blissful … excellent … if this is the promised cure to longevity then bring it on." – Emma Soames, *Daily Telegraph*

"I have not felt so good, so fast … " – Uma Thurman, *Red* magazine

"The Mayr clinic has given me my life back—or maybe just shown me my life. Thank you all." – Sarah Ferguson, Duchess of York, *Daily Telegraph*

"Delivers results fast … after six days … I have lost five pounds and my skin is clear." – Carolyn Asome, *The Times*

"If it's your life's ambition to be thin, hotfoot it to the original Mayr clinic where it all began … " – *Tatler* magazine

"Reader … take my word for it, Mayr & More can stand by its well-deserved reputation." – *Finch's Quarterly Review*

"I felt amazing—lighter, fresher and more energetic than I had in ages … And the great news is that the good feelings just kept getting better. By the end of the week, I had lost four pounds … and more came off in the weeks after I got back." – *Good Housekeeping*

"I've been given a new lease on life; energy at fifty that I didn't have at forty." – Angela Trainer, *Healthy Living* magazine

"Without trivializing the methodology, which works, it seems like common sense. Most of us eat too fast, too much and too late." – Jay Yeo, *Financial Times*

First published in North America in 2014 by
Harlequin Enterprises Ltd.
225 Duncan Mill Road
Don Mills, Ontario M3B 3K9
www.harlequin.com

Copyright © Elwin Street Productions 2014
Conceived and produced by
Elwin Street Limited
3 Percy Street
London W1T 1DE
www.elwinstreet.com

A CIP catalogue record for this book is available from the British Library
ISBN 978 03738 9300 3
10 9 8 7 6
Printed in China

Disclaimer: The advice, recipes and meal plans in this book are intended as a
personal guide to healthy living. However, it is not intended to provide medical
advice and it should not replace the guidance of a qualified physician or other
professional. Decisions about your health should be made by you and your
health-care provider based on the specific circumstances of your health, risk
factors, family history and other considerations. See your health-care provider
before making major dietary changes or embarking on an exercise program,
especially if you have existing health problems, medical conditions or chronic
diseases. The author and publishers have made every effort to ensure that the
information in this book is safe and accurate, but they cannot accept liability
for any resulting injury or loss or damage to either property or person, whether
direct or consequential and howsoever arising.

Reprinted by permission: as quoted on page 1

Seven Pillars of Health, Dr Don Colbert, January 2007, Siloam, Charisma House, Florida.

Crazy Sexy Diet, Kris Carr, December 2011, Skirt!, Globe Pequot, Guilford, Connecticut.

All rights reserved.

THE
ALKALINE
CURE

DR. STEPHAN DOMENIG

Medical Director, The Original F.X. Mayr & More Health Center

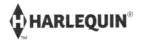

CONTENTS

Section 4: Preparing To Go Alkaline

Section 5: The Fourteen-Day Alkaline Cure

Section 6: The Recipes

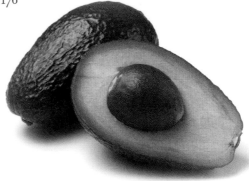

INTRODUCTION

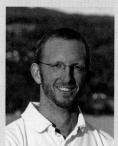

Dr. Stephan Domenig
Medical Director, the Original
F.X. Mayr & More Health Center

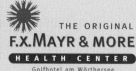

THE ORIGINAL
F.X. MAYR & MORE
HEALTH CENTER
Golfhotel am Wörthersee

I first studied medicine over twenty-one years ago. I was interested in people—why they behave the way they do, how they function and how and why they might be healthy or not. That last question was really the most difficult. Medical school told me everything I wanted to know about diseases and illnesses from a genetic or biochemical standpoint but there was nothing about what it means to be healthy. Everything was focused on illness. I wanted to know what makes us feel good but that was just not on the curriculum. The medicine I was taught was a downhill ski run all the way until you died. There was no going back.

Food was not mentioned. Neither was exercise. No one seemed interested in discovering the soul of an illness. I was fascinated by the more holistic approaches—the beauty of the whole body—and I was inspired by ancient health promoting techniques like Qi Gong and yoga. Medicine, for me, had to be more than just cutting up bodies and tying up bandages.

When I worked in geriatrics it was all about prolonging life, not the quality of that life. If someone reached one-hundred years old it was celebrated as a big success, never mind that they might not have gotten out of bed in fifteen years.

Then, over in the metabolical diseases (internal medicine) department there were a few pills and machines that could alleviate patients' suffering in the short term, but those methods were not what I would call medicine. There were very few attempts at understanding or trying anything different.

My first escape from this came with an inspiring course in chiropractics. There, I could use my hands to feel and touch the diseases—realign the spine, improve joint movements. This was fine at the time but I was still not treating the whole body. Then a friend gave me a book written in 1921 called *Fundamentals of the Diagnosis of Digestive Illnesses* by Dr. Franz Xaver Mayr.

Mayr explained very elegantly the complete physiology of digestion, its central role for well-being and the connection between tissue tone and function, inner health and posture as one way to evaluate health. It was the first explanation that seemed right in principle—in medicine. I trained to become a Mayr-doctor. I have now worked and treated thousands of patients. We combine old knowledge with a modern understanding of the body's biochemistry, its needs for certain nutrients and how what we eat and the way that we eat fundamentally influence our health.

Our approach to well-being centers around one keyword—balance. In the muscles, it's tension and relaxation. For food, it's alkaline and acid on a ratio of 2:1.

The modern Western diet, the ways we choose to eat and our lifestyles tend to encourage an acid overload—high stress jobs, high intensity exercise, and last but not least, high protein diets. Finding our way back to equilibrium is a great chance to improve overall health. That's what the cure is all about.

Our two-week program is a starting point, an introduction to being your own doctor. It is one that has helped a great many people. And it will help you, too.

Stephan Domenig
Lake Wörthersee, Austria

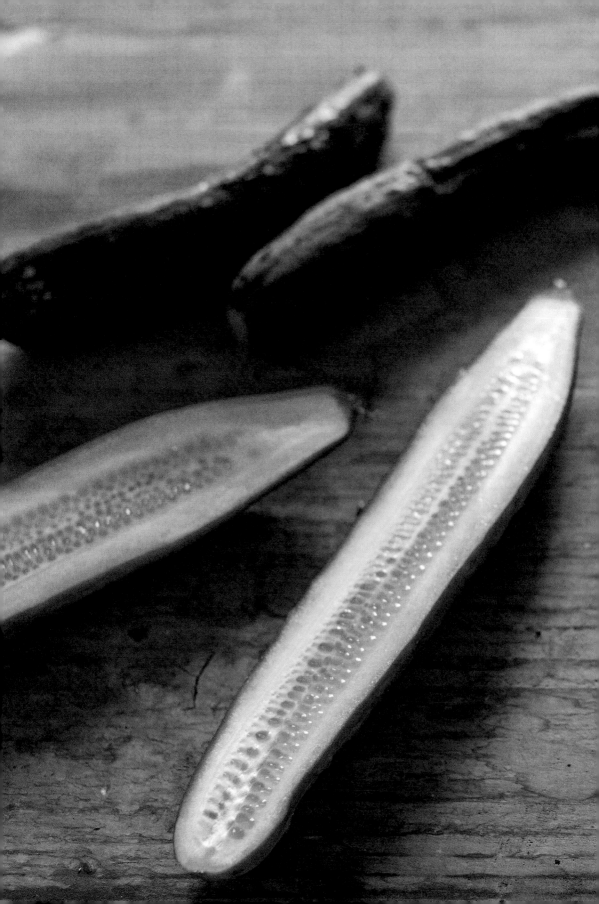

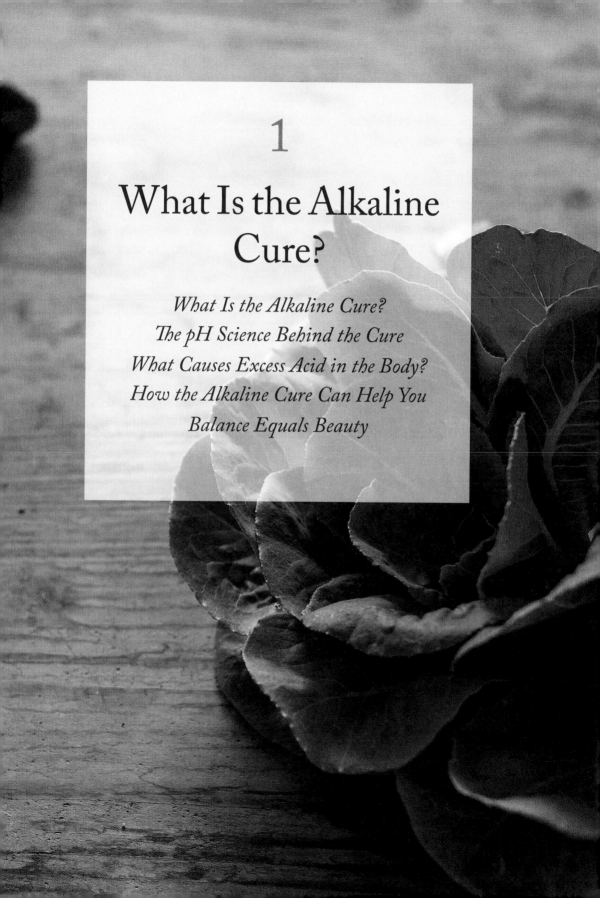

1

What Is the Alkaline Cure?

WHAT IS THE ALKALINE CURE?

The Alkaline Cure is a holistic approach to health and well-being. It is a set of simple but powerfully effective diet and lifestyle principles that will bring your digestive system into balance and your body back to its naturally healthy state. These are principles that anyone can follow.

How often do you eat quickly or on the run or late in the evening? And how often do you feel tired, lacking in energy and with a gassy, bloated stomach? These are sure signs your body is suffering from too much acid. The Alkaline Cure is the solution. It will recharge you, and it will reset your metabolism so that you can enjoy the energy levels you used to.

The benefits of the cure are both marked and swift. Regardless of your age and general level of health, if you follow the principles and the plan we give you in this book, you will begin to see results within two weeks. And, uniquely, you will be able to check those results yourself with the pH test papers we supply at the back of this book.

The cure is a powerful anti-aging program that will transform you from the inside out. The first benefits tend to be weight loss, increased vitality and improved complexion, skin tone and hair luster—which is why it is often been called a beauty cure. It will also reward you with stronger bones, better moods, enhanced brain function and a stronger immune system.

The Alkaline Cure is not a weight-loss program, although that may be one of its most popular benefits. We want you to find your natural, healthy body weight. Your body wants to be healthy; it used to be healthy. We can achieve that by cleaning our system of toxins and identifying the foods and habits that will help us perform better.

WHERE IT ALL BEGAN

For more than one hundred years, the teachings laid down by the great Dr. Franz Xaver Mayr have formed the basis of one of the most effective diet and health regimes in Europe. In that time, Mayr doctors have successfully treated tens of thousands of patients. Mayr, who was born in Austria in 1875, pioneered a radical new approach to wellness.

One of Mayr's pupils, Dr. Eric Rauch, opened the first Mayr health center in Dellach, on Lake Wörthersee in Austria, which is now known as the Original F.X. Mayr & More Health Center. It has been much admired, much copied and is a source of help to many people.

The Alkaline Cure has evolved through the study and research begun by Dr. F. X. Mayr. It is based on a clinical understanding of the effects different foods have on our digestive system. In the Mayr philosophy we believe that good digestion is the most important factor in human health. It is a holistic and preventative approach, which is to say it is not focussed on treating any one disease, but keeping the whole body healthy.

The alkaline approach has evolved over the years as the study of nutrition has shown us new ways to understand how our bodies deal with the foods we eat. However, the basic principles today, which we detail in section 3, remain the same as delineated by Dr. Mayr. We believe in the science of nutrition; we know that the food we eat and how we eat it can transform our performance.

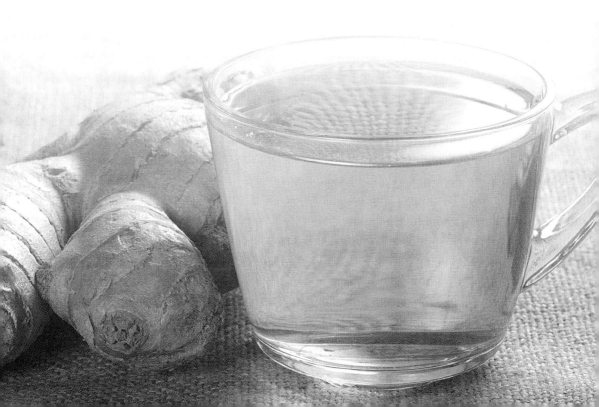

THE PH SCIENCE BEHIND THE CURE

As every farmer knows, you cannot get high yields from a field with acidic (or sour) soil. Just as in nature, so for the human body. At the Original F.X. Mayr & More Health Center we know that in order for the body to be healthy, it needs to have an acid-alkaline balance. How do we know this?

One of the most important methods we use at the health center for evaluating your health is testing your body's pH—in other words, whether your body is acid or alkaline, using the same pH scale that is used by doctors around the world. It is the only single test that gives us an indication of the general health of your body and its systems because the pH of your body's fluids, especially your blood, affects every cell in the body. Keep your body's pH in balance and you will stay healthy.

The beauty of using pH to evaluate health, is that it's as simple as reading numbers. Numbers for pH range from 1 to 14. The higher the pH number the more alkaline you are; 7 is considered neutral and anything below that becomes increasingly acidic. Although 7 is the neutral reading, for optimal health you should be slightly alkaline— ideally around 7.4. This is to counter the increase in acidity that comes with aging and diet.

Be Your Own Doctor

We have provided fourteen test papers and the pH chart at the back of the book to test your body's pH during the cure. We suggest you test yourself on a daily basis at home every morning shortly after you wake up and before eating anything. Don't worry if your initial readings are below 6 and towards the acid end. After two weeks of the cure you will notice a marked improvement. If your reading is already close to 7, that's great. You should still test yourself every day to track changes. Don't be tempted to test yourself more often than daily.

If you would like more test strips you can order these online from Micro Essential Inc. (www.microessentiallab.com).

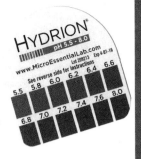

USING THE STRIPS

You can test your body's pH by using the strips with your saliva or your urine. It will take longer for the alkalizing effect of the cure to reach your urine, so you can generally expect a higher alkaline reading from your saliva. However, testing your urine will give you a more accurate reading as it is a better indicator of how well your kidneys are eliminating acid.

Saliva

The pH of your saliva is affected by what you have eaten or drunk recently. It is best to wait about two hours after a meal before you test, and then activate and swallow saliva several times to "rinse" the mouth.

Spit some saliva onto a spoon and wipe the litmus paper in the liquid, then compare the colored results with the chart in the packet.

Urine

The pH of your urine is affected by how much water you have consumed and the levels of acid-forming foods you have eaten. For this, it is best to test urine first thing in the morning.

Urinate a little into a cup and dip the litmus paper in quickly. Compare the colored results with the chart in the packet.

WHAT CAUSES EXCESS ACID IN THE BODY?

Our metabolism requires our digestive system to convert (digest) foods appropriately in order to absorb and utilize individual nutrients. Unhealthy eating habits—eating more food than our digestive system can handle at any one time—cause impaired digestion, which also impacts our acid-alkaline balance.

If your pH reading is lower than 7 then it means your body has excess acid. Excess acid in the body is called acidosis. Acidosis occurs when your kidneys and lungs can't keep your body's pH in check (see section 2). Acidosis is much more dangerous than excessive alkalinity (called alkalosis). That's why we are focused here on how to prevent and reduce excess acidity.

Both the foods you eat and how you eat them may give rise to excess acidity. The way a western diet has evolved in recent decades means many or, perhaps, most of us eat too much of the wrong kinds of foods (and drink the wrong drinks) with the result that they just clog up our systems and weigh us down.

Lifestyle habits are also a factor, including issues such as stress, lack of sleep, pollution and over-exercising (which causes lactic acid to form). The other major contributor to increasing acidity is age.

PREMATURE AGING AND ACIDITY

Sagging skin, stiff joints, muscle aches, chronic disease, cognitive deterioration, osteoporosis—we have come to accept these things as a part of growing old, but actually many of these problems are signs that your body is becoming too acidic.

Our modern lifestyles and diets cause us to age faster because we're forcing our bodies to deal with excess acid. In an acidic environment, our cells perform less efficiently and are unable to get rid of toxins. As well, many health issues are caused by acidic environments: it is a long list that includes irritable bowel syndrome, cardiovascular diseases, chronic fatigue, candida, histamine, gluten and other food allergies, diabetes and obesity.

SIGNS THAT YOUR BODY IS TOO ACIDIC

To a trained Mayr doctor, the symptoms of an acidic diet are easy enough to read. These everyday complaints are likely to be symptoms of an acidic diet. Do any of these sound familiar?

Constipation and bloating: both are caused by eating too fast, too much and/or overly acidic meals.

Lack of energy and focus: acid depletes blood oxygen availability and you feel sluggish as your brain and systems are deprived of this vital element.

Weight problems: being overweight suggests that your diet is incompatible with your body's ability to deal with the food it's given.

Poor complexion and dry, dull, lifeless skin: excess acid is eliminated through the skin, causing skin corrosion and inflammation.

Gum disease, tooth decay and bad breath: these can be directly related to a high-acid diet, allowing bacteria to develop much more quickly.

Frequent colds and flu: when the body is not being fed the right foods and the flora of the stomach changes, a weak immune system results.

Muscle and joint pains: inflammation can be a sign that the alkaline minerals in your bones and muscles are being extracted to neutralize acidity. Particular acids, like arachidonic acid, which is found in red meat, also trigger inflammation.

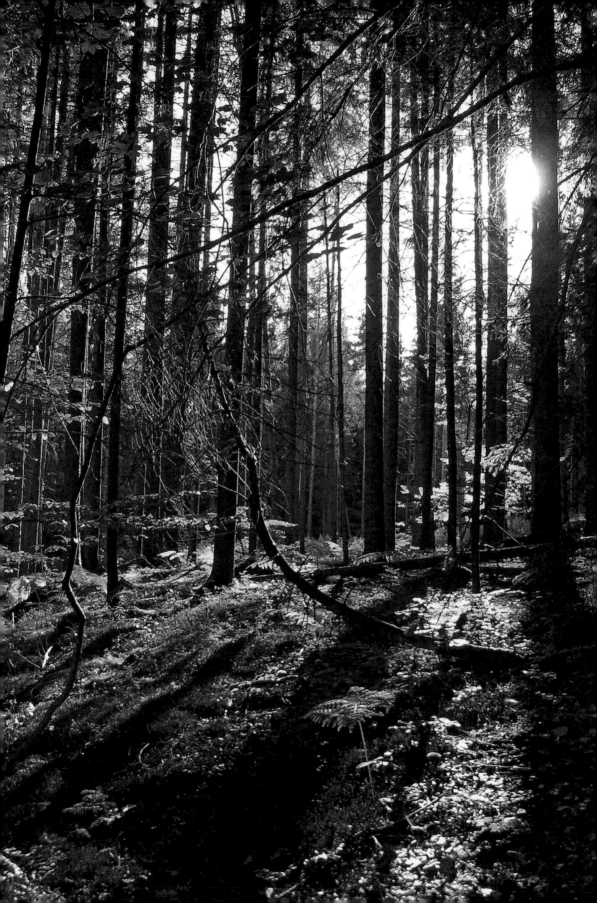

Since our bodies' acidity is affected by what we eat and how we live, we need to make diet and lifestyle changes to alkalize ourselves and stay healthy. The single most effective change you can achieve—and the aim of the Alkaline Cure—is to re-balance your diet by increasing your intake of alkaline foods so that two-thirds of everything you eat on the plate is alkaline and only one-third is acid. We are looking for foods that taste good, that complement each other and that are easy for your body to digest, so you maximize your performance. We are looking for foods that give you good health.

The 2:1 Alkaline to Acid Rule

In order to improve your alkalinity we do
not suggest only eating alkaline foods. The
best acid-alkaline balance of foods to aim for is two
parts alkaline to a maximum of one part acid. Ideally
this 2:1 ratio should be on your plate at every meal.
Realistically, this ratio is what you should bear in
mind over the course of your daily and weekly diet.
Be mindful, not fanatical.

Acid in Your Diet

We can classify all the food we eat as either acid-forming or alkaline-forming, meaning the foods release an acid or alkaline residue during the process of digestion. Note that foods that have an acidic taste (such as lemon, vinegar, rhubarb, etc.) are not necessarily acid-forming. So lemon, while acidic to taste, once digested actually has an alkalizing effect on the body. During the book, when we describe foods as "acid" or "alkaline" we will mean acid-forming or alkaline-forming.

The majority of acid-forming foods are basic staples (see page 67). The more we eat of these foods, the greater the production of acids. The situation can become harmful if the consumption reaches such a level that the metabolism is completely overburdened. There are many different kinds of acid-forming foods and their strength varies from strong to weak. The strongest acids are found in animal proteins as well as alcohol, caffeine, processed foods and sugar. The weakest acids are found in vegetable proteins, such as beans.

Alkaline-forming foods contain very little to no acid and do not produce any acids either. Alkaline foods include most vegetables, many fruits, cold-pressed oils, many grains and all herbs. However, the way we process/digest our food also impacts the effect on the body. If we eat something alkaline but rush and don't chew properly it ends up badly digested and ferments, causing acidity.

You can find tables on acid and alkaline foods in section 4.

The Problem of Protein

Protein is a macro-nutrient composed of amino acids that is necessary for the proper growth and function of the human body. Unfortunately, protein is also one of the most acidic foods, especially animal protein such as meat and fish (and certain types of cheese). On average, Americans eat about two-hundred pounds of meat a year, which is over twice more than the United States Department of Agriculture recommends. Most of us (except for serious athletes) eat far too much protein and our bodies become protein- and, therefore, acid-saturated. High-protein diets bring with them too much acidity for your stomach to cope with. They may help you lose weight in the short term but will destroy the body's acid/alkaline balance.

A Note on Calories

Over many years different foods have been blamed for making us fat, correctly or not. The whole conversation about diet has become overloaded with too many calorie counters. Because we look at diet from a different perspective and use the acid/alkaline monitor, calories are of less concern. Calories have their place and in a well-trained body they are burned off anyway. They only become an issue because we are sedentary and eat too much. Instead of counting calories you will be better off counting how many times you chew a mouthful of food.

HOW THE ALKALINE CURE CAN HELP YOU

One of the remarkable things about the Alkaline Cure is that while acidosis and its effects—the hardening of arteries, the clogging of the digestive system and other bodily malfunctions—may have been building up in your body over the course of many years, the process is swift to reverse. After you have learned the principles of the cure and followed the fourteen-day plan here, you will start to notice a difference. And friends and family will notice, too. But remember, the Alkaline Cure is a life plan, not a crash diet. It is one designed for the realization of optimal health.

The many benefits of the Alkaline Cure are extraordinary:

Slows Down the Signs of Aging
The primary and most rewarding benefit of the cure and one many of the other benefits below also contribute to. We don't promise to stop you aging but we do promise to keep you feeling and looking young and staying healthy. One reason that the Mayr Alkaline approach has often been labeled as a beauty treatment is that restoring alkalinity to the diet immediately eases many of our patients' skin, hair and nail problems. Skin regains its youthful radiance and elasticity, hair regains its sheen and nails stop being so brittle. We can rightly say the Alkaline Cure is a clinically-tested anti-aging plan.

Renews Energy and Vitality
You will experience renewed vitality as your metabolism improves. Digesting processed, protein-heavy, acid-forming foods requires energy, but without giving back the energy and nutrients it used to process the food. The result is lethargy.

Redressing the acid/alkaline balance corresponds with increased energy as cells pass oxygen around the body and restore vitality. An alkaline diet stabilizes energy levels through the day, avoiding the highs and lows of sugar rushes from acidic sources such as coffee or refined sugar. By regulating your eating times and changing your diet, you will also feel more energized because you will be sleeping better and deeper.

Encourages Weight Loss

You will lose weight—or, more importantly, find your natural body weight or Body Mass Index (BMI). Strictly, this is not a slimming diet. It works as a slimming diet because many of us are overweight, but our aim is a healthier you, a better functioning you, a more capable you. Your clearer digestive system and efficient metabolism will lead to weight loss as you clear the toxic load you have been carrying. Your renewed energy will also motivate you to exercise more so you will become fitter.

Reduces Bloating and Constipation

You will be able to go to the bathroom regularly and in comfort because you are working with your body, not against it. One very positive sign of good health is having clear urine and soft feces. Constipation is bad for you as it stresses your system. An alkaline diet is better than any laxative. If you eat well, you will go to the bathroom every morning. If you drink enough your stools will be softer. If you chew properly then the pressure on your stomach to perform is eased.

Improves Mood and Brain Function

Your mood will improve and you will start to feel more positive and less stressed. In 1987, Rudolph Wiley (PhD), conducted a study in which he postulated that acid imbalance contributes substantially, and often entirely, to disorders routinely classified as psychological, stress-related, psychosomatic or psychogenic. His study found that an alkaline diet reduced and eliminated the symptom severity in more than 85% of participants.

A broader choice of properly digested food should reduce peaks and troughs in amino acids and vitamins. Without vitamins like B6 (from fresh herbs, nuts, legumes, fish) you will get moody and have sleeping troubles. We also encourage work-life balance, taking gentle exercise, and avoiding alcohol, caffeine and processed food.

In addition to alleviating physical and mental stress, the Alkaline Cure will help support brain function because it encourages you to eat a diverse range of vitamin- and mineral-rich foods.

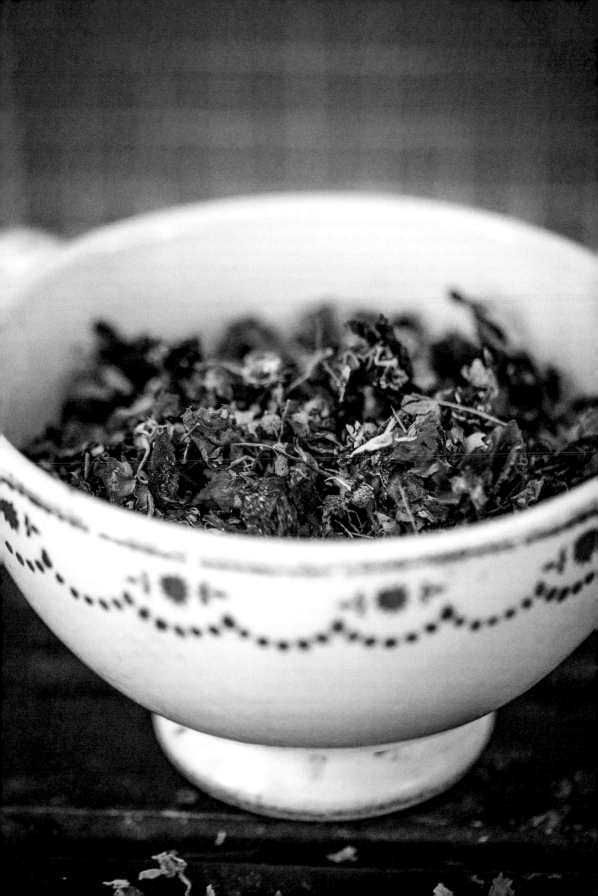

Defends Against Allergy and Disease

Many of our modern-day food allergies are actually an inflammation in the stomach. We see this increasingly in the health center where patients react badly to the gluten in wheat and the histamine in aged foods, milk proteins and, most dramatically, peanuts. Our treatment is to identify and avoid the aggravating foods and cleanse the system, giving it a rest from digesting large amounts of food and supplementing with alkalizing treatments.

Going beyond allergies, there is compelling scientific research linking diet and the prevalence of chronic disease such as cancer, heart disease and diabetes. Some theories suggest that these diseases thrive in an acidic environment and are suppressed by an alkaline environment. Additionally, alkaline foods such as vegetables and ripe fruits provide antioxidants, which are a first line of defense against these serious diseases. In essence, the healthier your stomach, the healthier your immune system.

Strengthens Bones

With the Alkaline Cure, you may find that muscular and skeletal pains start to ease. An alkaline diet can also help prevent and even treat osteoporosis as we reduce acidity and support our bones with alkalizing minerals. Overall, healthy bones require an alkaline atmosphere, vitamin D, calcium and weight-bearing exercise.

Increases Fertility

When your body is alkaline and not swamped with acid, the hormonal system slots back into its normal functionality which, in many cases we have seen, leads to much greater fertility in men and women. An alkaline environment guarantees better cell function. Many patients at the clinic who thought they could not have children go on to conceive shortly after completing the cure.

BALANCE EQUALS BEAUTY

The Alkaline Cure is a simple equation. Regulating your acid-alkaline balance is an integral part of your overall health. Your body needs a balance of alkaline and acid foods, in a ratio of two-thirds alkaline and one-third acid, so that overall you are slightly alkaline. Combining acidic and alkaline foods at every meal is the ideal but may not be realistic. If you have eaten a lot of acidic food on an evening out, have an alkaline day the next day to compensate. The key to long-term health is about making small adjustments and developing healthy habits. It really is simple. It really is effective.

Philosophy of Nutrition

The Alkaline Cure is not a fad diet. There are no calorie counters or gimmicks. It is not about going hungry or going vegetarian, although we do recommend that you eat more vegetables. It isn't strictly a diet at all because it is not about weight loss at the expense of your overall health. The Alkaline Cure is about exchanging bad habits for good ones. It is a philosophy of nutrition that will ensure good health and weight loss (if your body needs it). That's why we call it a cure not a diet.

The Alkaline Cure is a medically proven approach, based on scientific knowledge from the Original F.X. Mayr & More Health Center, which has evolved successfully over many decades. It contains everything you need to achieve and maintain balance and vitality in your life and it will restore your body back to its naturally healthy state. For which it will thank you.

It is your body. Be nice to it. Its fate is in your hands.

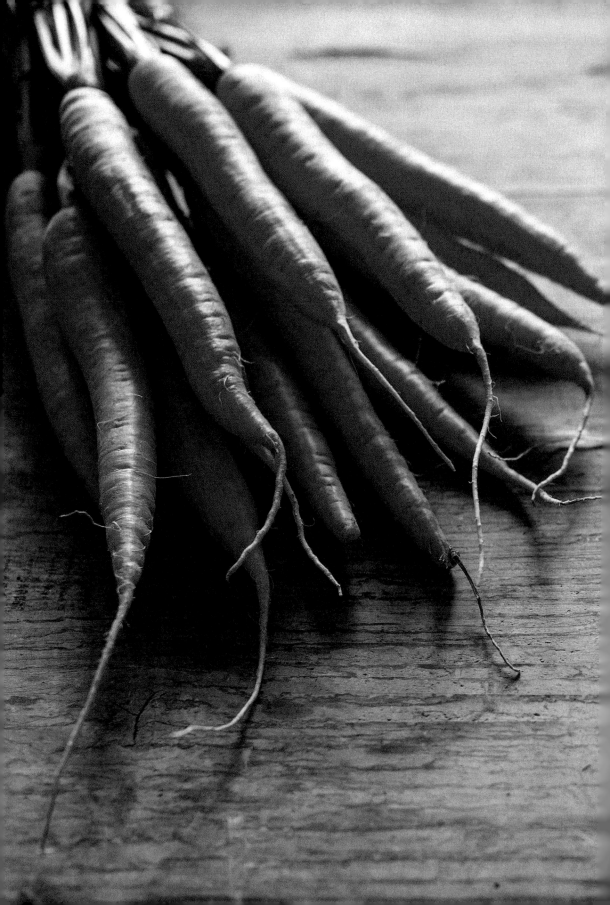

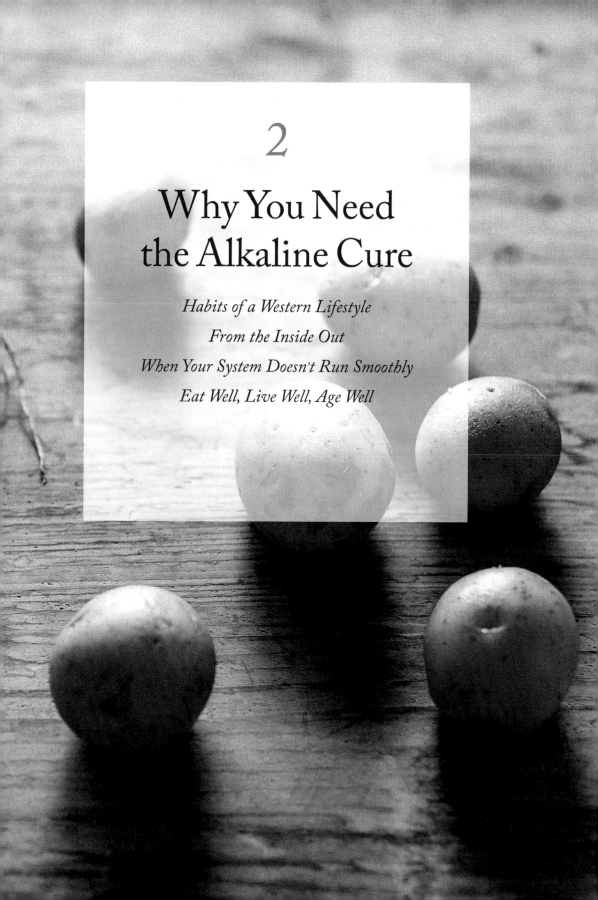

2

Why You Need the Alkaline Cure

Habits of a Western Lifestyle

From the Inside Out

When Your System Doesn't Run Smoothly

Eat Well, Live Well, Age Well

HABITS OF A WESTERN LIFESTYLE

The Western world is getting fatter. Two-thirds of the American population is overweight, and half that number is considered obese. Diabetes rates are at an all-time high—an estimated 25.8 million people in the United States have diabetes.

Take a stroll down any urban main street and the signs and symptoms are there. We are getting bigger. And despite advances in modern medicine, we are still plagued by chronic disease. Most worryingly our children are getting bigger and facing a future of widespread health problems. Currently, one in three children is overweight, and the Center for Disease Control and Prevention predicts that one in three children born after the year 2000 will develop diabetes at some point in their life. Furthermore, one in twenty children under five will develop at least one food allergy.

In a sense we have forgotten how to eat: we eat too much, we eat the wrong foods, we eat at the wrong times. Overall, we consume too much meat, fish and sugar. We buy too many refined and processed foods that simply fill us up without delivering any real value to help our bodies function. Too much of what we eat has no nutritional value at all—it has been stripped of nutrition through processing before it even gets to us.

Stressing the Diet

The stresses of modern life have encouraged us to see foods as something they are not and to overlook their essential medicinal qualities. Technology has altered the basic things we used to take for granted and depend on, such as bread. We no longer shop at bakers, butchers and fishmongers in local shops where people know what they are selling. Rather, we shop in box stores and supermarkets where no one is too sure what they are selling us.

It may sound like a contradiction to say that something like white bread is now so denatured that it does not deliver any nutritional value and yet it still fattens us. It is just empty calories, taking up the space in the stomach where other more useful foods could take its place.

Invisible Changes

Overly acidic meals change the shapes of our bodies, which may stop us from exercising properly. Visibly, we become fatter. But that is just a symptom with its own impact on our health: weighing down our ability to perform physically, overstressing our frames and creating problems in our skeletons. What starts with aches and pains can lead to hip and knee replacements. We become immobilized.

The less visible change is what is happening inside our bodies. Before we get fat, our bones demineralize, our skin sags from lack of nutrients and the toxins we struggle to deal with put strain on our systems. We cope, but we are losing our vitality, our energy, our health.

Toxin Overload

Too much acidity makes us age quicker. Worse, being too acidic creates an environment in the body where allergies and diseases can flourish. Our digestive tract naturally tries to balance out the mixture of things we consume. The problem is that too much of what we eat is acid-forming and too little is alkaline-forming.

Recovering an Alkaline Balance

How we eat is as important as what we eat. In a busy, modern world the danger is that we are often grabbing food on the go or squeezing meal times into short gaps and this serves to overload the digestive system. When we eat too quickly we do not give our bodies the chance to digest food fully and absorb the nutrients.

The way our diets have evolved in recent decades—and many of these changes are quite recent—has altered us. What we are eating clogs up our systems and weighs us down. These foods stop us from performing at our best, and over time they even change the natural shape of our bodies altogether. We have become accustomed to thinking of everyday foods as healthy when much of what we eat has little nutritional value and just passes through us without delivering any of the minerals or vitamins we need.

Taking Active Steps Towards Health

The answer is not a simple pill, nor to eat more of one particular food. Diets that focus on one element—such as the cabbage soup diet or the fasting diet—miss the point. The essential goal should be to redress the overall imbalance. By focusing on how our bodies perform and feeding our bodies what they need, we can regain our strength.

In other words, if we cut down on the acid-forming foods—which are largely the proteins, refined fats and sugars we have become accustomed to—and replace them with more alkalizing foods, we can take active steps towards changing our health.

If we change what and how we eat then we might not get ill in the first place. It is not simply the foods themselves that are at issue but also our body's ability to process them. We are often told that we should be eating a "balanced diet" without quite knowing what that really means.

If you follow the simple ratio of 2:1 alkaline foods to acid, you will achieve that balanced diet. You can revitalize your life by eating a healthier, less acidic, low-protein diet and establishing a positive balance between exercise and rest.

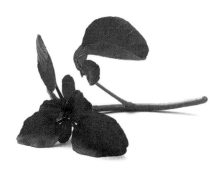

WELCOME TO ACID AMERICA

Let us take a look at the everyday American diet. The levels of acidity in each of these meals is going to lurch your pH to the wrong end of the scale. Unfortunately, this is what the average American has been eating.

BREAKFAST

Scrambled eggs with toast, sausages, orange juice and a coffee with milk and sweeteners.

SNACK

A bagel and more coffee to keep you going.

LUNCH

It's lunch time and you are hungry again. You buy a cheeseburger and fries. You wash each big bite down with a gulp of soda and check your emails on your phone so that this lunch isn't "wasted." Greasy, tasty, "satisfying"— you're full, so you must be nourished, right? Wrong.

SNACK

Sitting at your desk, focused on your mountain of work, you start feeling a bit lethargic—you need something for energy. Grab a candy bar and a soda for a fast pick-me-up.

DRINK WITH FRIENDS

You grab a couple of martinis with the boss on the way home; more empty calories, more acidity.

DINNER

You get home from work, exhausted. You just want something quick and filling: a chicken breast, fried, with a fluffy white dinner roll on the side. Finish the night with several glasses of wine and something sweet. Good night. But you probably won't sleep well.

FROM THE INSIDE OUT

Your nutrition affects everything about you—how fast you age, the quality of your skin, your organs, your energy levels and productivity, your mood and emotions, your weight and, on a grander scale, whether chronic disease will thrive in your body. It has a powerful impact on your quality of life.

At the Original F.X. Mayr & More Health Center, we believe the digestive system is at the center of health and well-being. Its role is to process the food we give it—good or bad. The better it functions, the better we function, and the better we look and feel. Nutritionists sometimes talk about a stomach having its own brain. Eating is the last voluntary mental act we can decide on. After that our body takes over and decides for itself what it is going to do.

A DAY IN THE LIFE OF YOUR DIGESTIVE SYSTEM

Digestion is the process of breaking down food so that nutrients can be absorbed and used by cells, tissues, organs and systems. A healthy digestive system sets up a rhythm for the day. Each twenty-four hour cycle should, ideally, start with a good breakfast and end the next morning in the bathroom. We are all different so the cycle can vary according to what we have eaten and our personal metabolisms.

The Importance of Enzymes

Enzymes are protein-based molecules that start, control and terminate every biochemical process in our bodies, such as digesting proteins and fats, breaking down and eliminating toxins, neutralizing acids, converting food into energy for cells, and extracting amino acids from food to build our DNA. There are three categories of enzymes: metabolic (these run each organ and system in our bodies), digestive and food enzymes. Each organ has different enzymes that require specific pH environments to function optimally.

The Role of Saliva

The process of digestion starts in the mouth where chewing and saliva start to break down starch and protein. Chewing is important for different reasons. Firstly, it allows us to taste and enjoy our food. Secondly, in the act of chewing we generate more saliva, which is key for digestion. Thirdly, it warns the rest of the body that food is coming. And masticating and grinding up food, especially proteins like meat, makes it easier for the rest of the body to cope with what is coming. If we swallow our food down, or gulp it, or even wash it down with a glass of water, then we are asking our stomachs to do all the work, something they are not altogether designed to do.

Saliva helps to maintain a neutral pH in our mouths and provides a reservoir of calcium and phosphate ions to remineralize the teeth and prevent tooth decay. Saliva also contains enzymes that are essential to kickstarting the digestion of fats and starches, preparing them for processing in other parts of the digestive system. Longer chewing means longer exposure to these enzymes. Finally, saliva is bacteria's first contact with your immune system—if you bypass the mouth then you miss your body's first line of defense.

The Role of the Stomach

The stomach is a big acid cauldron that breaks down food as a necessary part of digestion. In order to digest food and kill the kinds of bacteria and viruses that come with it, the inside of our stomachs are acidic with a pH balance of around 1.5. The stomach uses acid and enzymes to break that food into pieces that are more easily digested in the next stage of the process—which happens in the small intestine.

Roughly speaking, most of us will retain food in our stomachs for anything from thirty minutes to four hours. However, different foods pass through the stomach—or get cleared to go to the next stage—at different speeds. Melon, for example, being nearly all water, might travel on quickly while a hunk of beef protein will be kept behind for extra processing. The stomach also produces sodium bicarbonate, which it sends out around the body. Sodium bicarbonate as well as other bicarbonates are called "alkaline buffers" and they help to neutralize excess acid in the body.

The Role of the Small and Large Intestines

An important change occurs in the digestive system between the stomach and the small intestine. The stomach is highly acidic, which it needs to be in order to break up the food mix. When it passes this acid mix down to the small intestine, your pancreas releases digestive juices that are highly alkaline and that neutralize the acids from the stomach. The juices are also rich in enzymes that further break down fats, proteins and carbohydrates.

The main roles of the small intestine are to chemically digest food and absorb nutrients. By the time the food leaves the small intestine, almost every nutrient from it has entered the bloodstream. The kidneys filter the blood and sieve out any excess water, toxins and acid waste. In order to keep the mix moving, it is important to drink plenty of fluids; generally speaking, the color of your urine will be darker if you are not drinking enough fluids and paler if you are drinking a lot. All that remains is passed to your large intestine for further processing.

In the large intestine, the last of the nutritional value is extracted. The major functions of the large intestine are to absorb water from the remaining indigestible food matter, absorb electrolytes, metabolize vitamins and amino acids and store and excrete waste from the body. The large intestine takes its time, which can be upwards of twelve hours. Once, or sometimes twice, a day it will end its shift and send a consignment down to the rectum for excretion.

Simplicity and Routine

Just as eating at regular times is good practice, so too is going to the bathroom at regular times. First thing in the morning is the most obvious time, although for some people it can take a few hours for the metabolism to get going after they wake up.

What our stomach wants is a regular life. Simple foods at the right time that don't make it work too hard. In treatments at the Original F.X. Mayr & More Health Center, we deliberately try to focus on a small range of foods that allow the stomach to reboot itself.

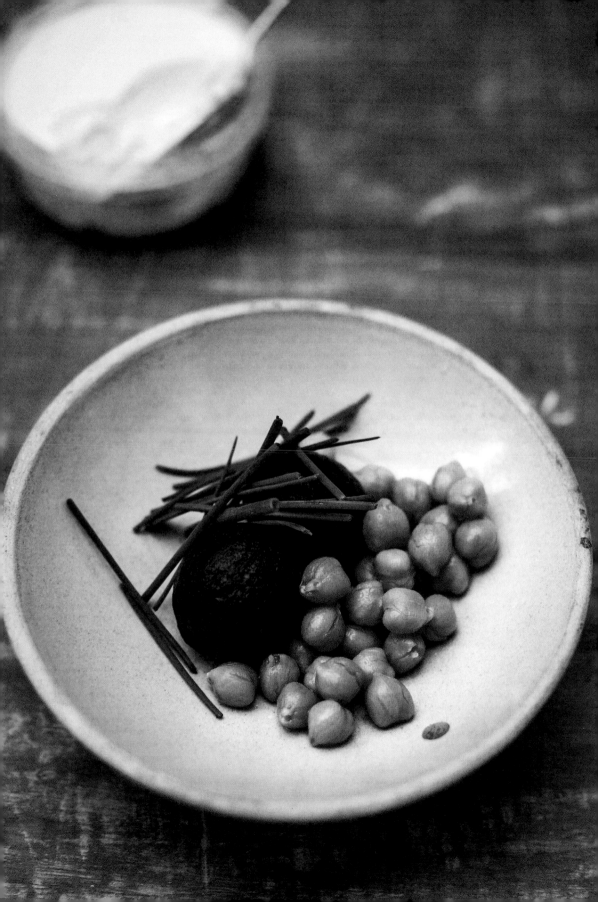

WHEN YOUR SYSTEM DOESN'T RUN SMOOTHLY

Your body is designed to run like an efficient machine but bad eating habits can wreak havoc on your digestive system. If you eat too fast or too much or too late—or all three—you can overload your digestive system and hamper your stomach's ability to digest.

FERMENTATION

A stomach can only hold and process so much food at a time. If there is more food than it can deal with the stomach sags and the excess food is left to putrefy and ferment, eventually moving on with only minor processing. This is made even worse if another batch of food comes along before the stomach is naturally ready. And if the food being digested is strongly acidic or is taken in late in the evening then the putrefaction is accelerated. As the resulting acids pass down the system they hamper the work of the enzymes that would otherwise translate the mixture into energy and nourishment. In other words, fermentation causes reduced digestive ability, which greatly impacts our overall health and well-being.

Usual physical manifestations of putrefaction and fermentation are gas, burping and bad breath. When people complain of heartburn, what they should be saying is stomach burn because that is what it is.

Elimination of Acids

Acids in our metabolism are eliminated mainly by the lungs and the kidneys. The carbon dioxide we exhale as we breathe is the quickest way to excrete acid; the alkaline buffers in the kidneys eliminate stomach acids via our urine. Our acid/alkaline balance depends to a large extent on whether these two organs are fulfilling their function of filtering and eliminating properly. Intracellular acidosis, a condition where your body fluids contain too much acid, occurs when your kidneys and lungs cannot keep your body's pH in balance because the enzymes struggle to digest the food and the alkaline buffers are unable to excrete the acids.

Strong Acids vs. Weak Acids

If the digestive system is overloaded with excess acids not only do the acids affect the body's cells and enzymes but also the body has to eliminate these acids in ways that can harm your health. Weak acids (from plant origins) are relatively easy to eliminate from the body by the usual methods. Stronger acids require more work by the kidneys, which have a limited capacity each day to do this, especially as you grow older. Two ways that the body deals with excess acid involves your skin and bones. Your body can eliminate excess acid through the skin and by sweating, which causes wrinkles, dryness and inflammation. Your body can also leach valuable minerals from your bones in order to neutralize the acids. By depleting the calcium and mineral reserves in your bones, the acids put you at greater risk of developing osteoporosis, which can, however, be prevented by calcium supplements, vitamin D and, most importantly, restoring your acid/alkaline balance through diet.

Acids clearly have a significant impact on the functionality of your whole body, but by redressing the acid/alkaline balance, we're certain you will reap the benefits of better-functioning organs, more beautiful and radiant skin and stronger bones.

Raw Vegetables

Raw vegetables and raw fruits are important alkaline contributors but they are especially prone to fermentation. If we eat most of our fruit and vegetables in their raw forms, we don't get the alkaline benefit and instead become more acidic. We can avoid this by staying away from raw foods in the evening and not eating more raw foods than our digestive system can properly digest.

THE EFFECTS OF STRESS

The stomach reacts very badly to stress of any kind—emotional or physical. It does not like it. It seizes up and stops functioning as efficiently. If you are eating while stressed, the stress signals tell your stomach you're doing something else. You are not eating. Your stomach reacts by hunkering down and waiting for things to get better.

Therefore eating when stressed is, nutritionally speaking, a bad idea. The stomach will either hang on to anything it has got or pass it on without doing its normal job. For the same reason eating on the run is also not a good idea. In both instances, only a modicum of the nutrients will be extracted.

Modern everyday pick-me-ups like cola, coffee and alcohol may seem like they help with stress but they don't. Sugar is the worst culprit, offering a short fix but then disappearing—leaving behind the calories, draining the body's minerals and making us crave for more.

AN AGING DIGESTIVE SYSTEM

As your body ages, it tends to have more digestive problems because natural supplies of enzymes decrease. Vital digestive processes start to slow and we get ill because acid toxins can't be eliminated efficiently, food isn't digested and absorbed properly and energy isn't delivered to our cells.

You may be able to cope with a soda and fries in your twenties, but over the years the accumulation becomes all too visible. You need a diet rich in alkaline foods that can replenish your enzyme stores and help your body combat the symptoms of aging.

This is just part of the evidence that helped F.X. Mayr, and those of us who followed him, understand that to be healthy and to have a well-functioning metabolism we need to have an efficient digestive system. And that includes eating the right balance of foods. Put simply, we know that if you eat well, you will live well and age well.

EAT WELL, LIVE WELL, AGE WELL

Modern medicine has achieved wonderful breakthroughs, but its achievements should not obscure or divert us away from a simple truth—if we pay attention to and carefully choose the foods we eat everyday, then we would not have to go to the doctor in the first place.

Eat Well

Franz Xaver Mayr's philosophy was to treat all his patients in the same way. He argued that if the stomach and the digestive system function properly, many diseases would not appear in the first place—a healthier body doesn't allow them to flourish.

The power of food to heal the human body is proven in front of our eyes every day at the health center. We see firsthand that patients lose weight. We also have seen patients—both men and women— who thought they could not conceive children but were able to do so after following the dietary advice here. Stomach pain eases and skin clears—these are immediate signs pointing to a healthier future. Also central to the Mayr approach is *how* we eat—chewing well and taking your time are crucial to good health.

The past decades have seen an unprecedented increase in fast food consumption and the industrialization of what we eat. More and more of our food is being processed and loaded with preservatives, flavor enhancers, added sugar and salt. These have a demonstrable ill-effect on our health and well-being. We need to return to natural, organic foods that are in season.

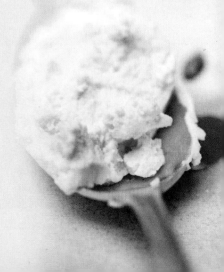

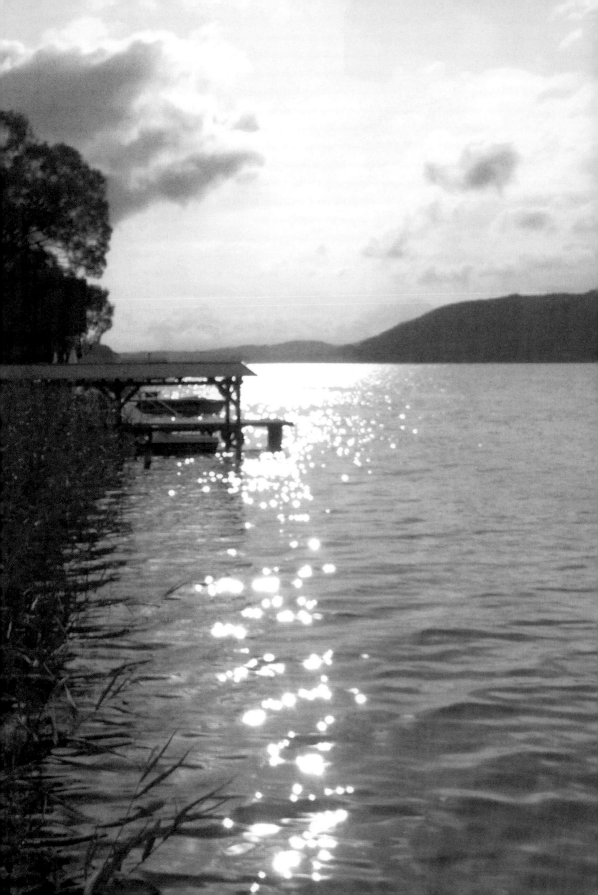

Live Well

However, diet alone is not the answer to good health. Another fundamental part of our approach is a better lifestyle. Gentle cardio and breathing exercises improve blood circulation, strengthen the body and, in turn, support the internal systems and ease stress. Activities that bring you joy—such as dancing, hiking, swimming—or peace—such as yoga or meditation—are also good for us.

Our immediate surroundings are important to our health. Open windows bring fresh air. Plants and flowers supply oxygen. Music soothes and brings happiness.

Age Well

We all grow old but acidic diets and poor lifestyle cause us to age faster than we naturally should. We have come to accept chronic ailments and diseases as a normal part of living. However, many symptoms of old age can be postponed by a healthier diet. Most diseases and ailments develop over years. A cup of coffee this morning is not going to kill you. A hamburger is not going to kill you. The long term effects of these acidic foods—for instance, the leaching of minerals from bones—happens slowly but builds up over years.

The Alkaline Cure will put your body back in harmony by eradicating these negative influences and encouraging a change in your eating and lifestyle. Life is always about balance, rhythm and cycles, and the only person who can tell you to take action is you.

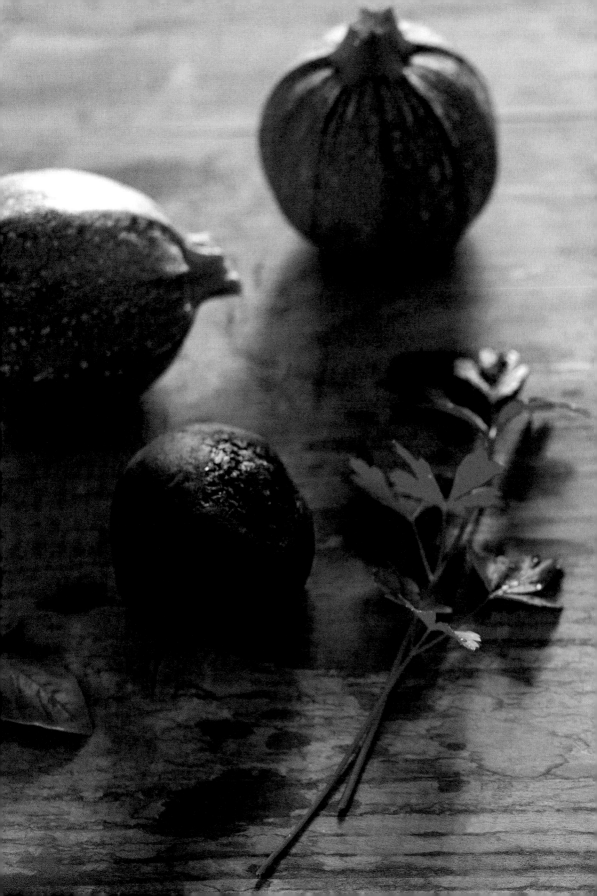

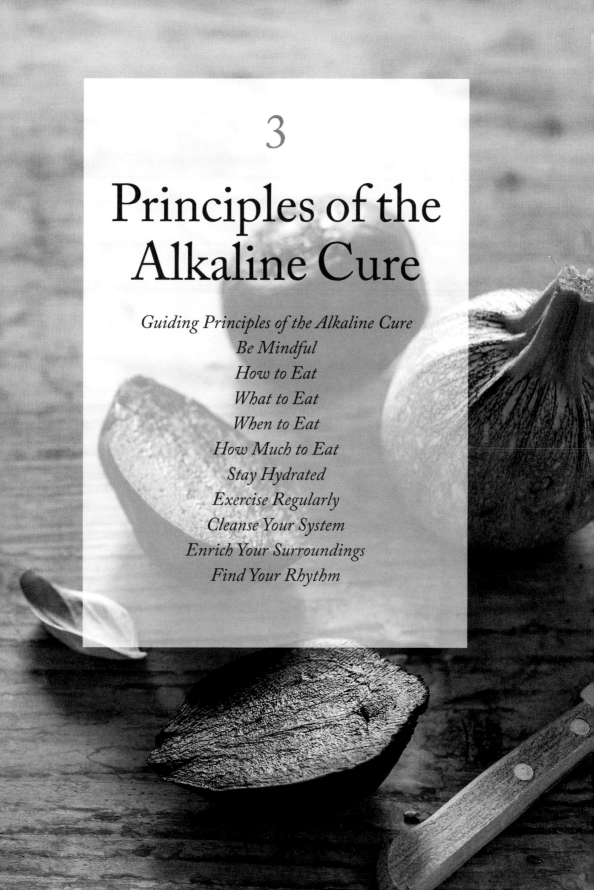

3
Principles of the Alkaline Cure

GUIDING PRINCIPLES
OF THE ALKALINE CURE

The Alkaline Cure is a prescription for health, designed to help pull your body out of its acidic state by balancing your acid/alkaline intake. Remember, you do not want to cut out all acid foods; instead you want to eat fewer acid foods and more alkaline ones to redress a long-instilled imbalance in your body's pH. You don't need to get off the couch and run a marathon; you need moderate and regular exercise. Your body doesn't want extremes—it wants balance.

It's important to pay attention to how you're eating and how you feel afterward. Do you rush meals so you can move on to something else? Do you only chew a few times and then swallow food almost whole? Do you wash your food down with a drink during a meal? Do you eat on the run? All of these have a bigger impact on your overall health than you realize.

Eating alkaline means breaking away from some of the accepted norms that you've grown accustomed to, particularly when it comes to portion size. Eating heavy acidic meals late at night really does harm your health. Quality of food and smaller portions should be the new norm—choosing fresh, local and seasonal foods and combining them in the 2:1 ratio.

The Alkaline Life

To reap the long-term benefits of the cure, we want to encourage you not to think just about the fourteen-day diet plan. This book should serve as a starting point for how to live alkaline. Let us introduce you to the ten principles we preach and practice at the Original F.X. Mayr & More Health Center, that will help guide you to healthy habits.

The first and most important principle is that of mindfulness, or what is sometimes called consciousness. The last principle echoes that philosophy by reminding us to find for ourselves the same regularity and rhythm in life that we can find in nature. This is the way to harmony and balance, not just in nutrition but in life.

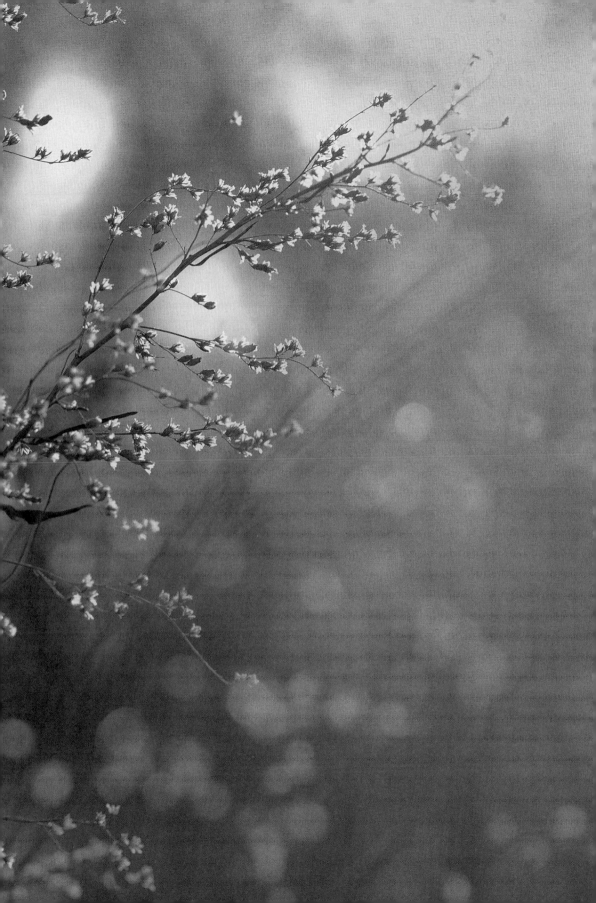

1. BE MINDFUL

Achieving long-term contentment, relaxation and general mental health is important if you want to lead a good-quality life. Stress, poor sleep and general unhappiness not only affect your day-to-day life, but they make your body more susceptible to illness and disease.

Balancing your body and your mind should start with awareness of how your body feels, how you respond emotionally to situations and your eating and lifestyle habits. It is about centering yourself, knowing yourself and being in calm control of yourself. There are techniques to help you develop good habits and a balanced lifestyle.

One method for balancing mind and body is MBSR (Mindfulness-Based Stress Reduction), a technique that helps prevent and treat burnout and stress-related illnesses. MBSR combines Buddhist meditation techniques and elements from yoga in a nonreligious/nonesoteric way in order to train the mind. The aim is to make awareness part of your daily routine. This involves conscious focus of attention to the moment with nonjudgmental awareness and perception of your body, emotions and environment. This heightened awareness should enable you to observe these things more clearly and realistically and regulate your emotions.

The Benefits of Mindful Eating

Many of us have come to view meals as a necessity that can be bashed out of the way to make time for doing other things, such as work, house chores or television. We regularly take meals on the run or at an office desk, and sometimes we even gulp down a plate of food at home—we move into autopilot and mechanically stab, chew and swallow. Even with healthy food, if we shovel it in quickly it doesn't get digested properly and stresses our systems. Mealtimes should be our own time, family time, a chance to anchor and be at one with the world. Considering how important food is to keeping us alive, we should give it more of our time. When we don't do that, we diminish our spirit, our nutrition. We won't always have time to do this, but erring toward this as often as possible is highly beneficial.

TEN STEPS FOR MINDFUL EATING

1. Give yourself time to eat. Each meal time should be no less than thirty minutes at the table.

2. Make sure you are comfortably seated. Take a couple of deep breaths to settle yourself and accept that this is time set aside for a meal. Be thankful that you have nutritious food to eat.

3. Notice any feelings of impatience and urges to get on and just eat the food. Perhaps you are thinking of things you need to do, but try to concentrate. This time is dedicated to enjoying your food.

4. Look at the food on your plate. Appreciate its visual qualities. Smell your food—breathe in the mouthwatering aromas.

5. Before you start to eat, think about how much food you put on your fork—the smaller, the better.

6. When you put the food in your mouth, take your time while chewing to appreciate the different flavors and textures.

7. Chew well, around thirty times is the minimum. Ensure the food in your mouth is fully masticated before you swallow.

8. Put your fork down between bites, it's important to take your time and rest so that you don't overwhelm your stomach.

9. Resist any urge to rush—perhaps on to dessert, to the next bite of food or to get up and do something else.

10. When you have finished, stay seated and relaxed for a few minutes. You should feel calm, satisfied and nourished, not bloated or overfull. Your body and your mind will thank you for taking the time.

2. HOW TO EAT

The first law of eating well is to take your time. Do not eat when you are stressed or angry, which might cause you to hurry. When you do eat, it's important to set aside enough time to give your body a chance to absorb what it is being fed, especially at breakfast and lunch. You need to relearn the pleasures of eating properly.

Your body digests different foods in different parts of the digestive tract and needs time to carry out this process. It should come as no surprise that your body will perform this task more efficiently when you are relaxed.

The Art of Chewing

Digestion starts in the mouth. Grinding food into smaller, softer parcels is going to help the gut process it better. If your food isn't chewed well enough, you may end up feeling bloated and flatulent since large food particles that pass through the stomach to the intestine attract more bacteria which can generate gas and discomfort.

Nutrient absorption is also affected by insufficient chewing and improper digestion. Chewing triggers your system to produce acids in the stomach, which break down the food so it can be absorbed. If you don't chew properly, other parts of the digestive system have to work harder to process the food, potentially making you feel lethargic.

Studies have shown that people who eat slower tend to eat less and are, therefore, less likely to be overweight. The longer you take to chew your food, the longer you will take to finish your meal. As you eat, a message is sent to the brain to indicate you are getting full. If you eat too fast, the brain will think you are still hungry, even though you have consumed enough calories. Rushing through a meal may also prevent you from really tasting your food, leading to you not feeling satisfied by it. By taking your time, you have a chance to enjoy the unique flavors, textures and colors of the foods on your plate.

Chewing your food properly—as many as fifty times according to F.X. Mayr—not only breaks down your food into digestible packets and better satisfies your appetite, but also brings your saliva into play.

An Exercise in Appreciating Food

The point of this raisin exercise, which we practice at the
health center, is to show how something as humble as a
raisin can teach us how to eat mindfully.

Take a raisin. Look at it carefully and smell it. Sense the
sweet smell spreading through your nose, filling you with
expectations of the taste. Put the raisin in your mouth and
feel it with your tongue. Now chew carefully: notice how
the taste spreads through your mouth. Observe how you
feel and decide when you're ready to swallow. All the energy
of the sun and the nutrients from the earth collected in that
little raisin are in you now. You will digest it perfectly. This
exercise should take about four minutes.

It is crucial that food spends sufficient time in the mouth to allow it to
mix properly with saliva, an important component in the digestive mix.
A healthy person produces three to six cups of saliva per day, which is
one reason why a glass of warm water is one of the best ways to start
the day. With some foods, chewing fifty times a mouthful can be more
difficult, but the process of mastication is beneficial even if it is a leaf
of lettuce, because the saliva that chewing induces prepares the rest of
the digestive system for what is about to happen.

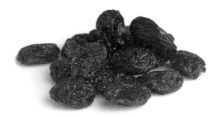

3. WHAT TO EAT

What you eat directly affects your alkaline/acid balance. As we mentioned earlier, the ideal alkaline to acid ratio is 2:1—meaning every acidic food on your plate should be paired with twice the amount of alkaline foods.

However, it's not just the type of food that you eat but also the quality of your food that has a significant impact on your health. The mineral profiles of vegetables are affected by factors such as the soil they are grown in, since that is where the vegetables themselves source their nutrition. Therefore, we encourage you to look for fresh, seasonal, local foods of the best quality to make sure that what you eat is worthwhile both gastronomically and nutritionally. Organic produce is generally better because if your food is grown using pesticides and fertilizers, it is going to be nutritionally depleted.

Eat from the Land Around You
Food always has more value when it comes from the land and sea around you. The greater the distance it has come, the more hands that will have touched it, and the more likely that it will have been processed or acidified along the way. In addition to freshness and quality, local also tends to mean smaller, craft businesses that contribute to your local economy. Generally, the larger the business, especially in the food industry, the larger the compromises that have been made...

Pick Food for Each Season
You want foods at the peak of their ripeness, when they contain a maximum amount of nutrients. This is especially true of fruit. Our lives are rhythmical and we should follow the changes as they happen. Supermarkets tend to make us believe there is only one season, where everything is available all the time. This is a myth. Depending on where you live, strawberries may be ripe in July, plums in September, apples in October, beets in November. Markets and small shops also let you buy one or two vegetables at a time to get a good mix—multipacks of fruit and vegetables tend to overwhelm the shopping basket and the refrigerator.

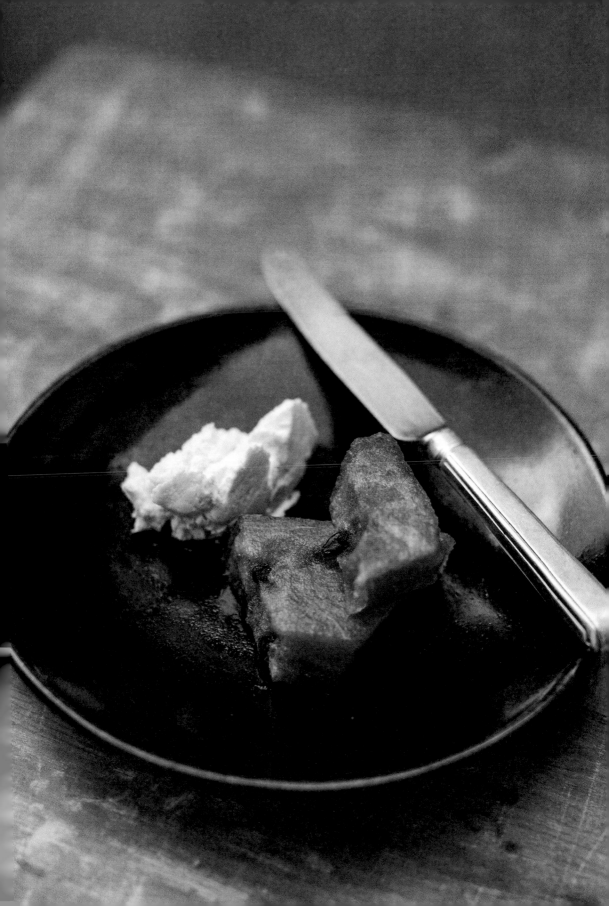

4. WHEN TO EAT

Make the most important meals of the day breakfast and lunch. When you wake in the morning your body is at its most able, in a digestive sense. It can cope with a wide range of different foods more easily. In the evening, though, your body, like you, is slowing down, so you are looking for smaller portions of more digestible foods. The habit of eating substantial meals later in the evening is not good from a digestive point of a view. Evening meals should be consumed early, preferably before six in the evening, since eating late can have several effects including:

* **Sleep deprivation:** your body's rhythms are programmed to complete the digestive process within twenty-four hours. Eating late disrupts this rhythm. Your body starts to slow down after sunset, preparing for sleep at nightfall. During sleep, your body and your digestive system need a break to cleanse and prepare for the next day. If you eat a meal as your body is winding down in the evening, then your metabolism is forced to gear up to digest the food, using energy while you sleep. This activity can result in poor sleep and lethargy.

* **Acid reflux:** when you eat a meal and then lie down to sleep, your horizontal orientation may allow acid from your stomach to travel up the esophagus, which can cause inflammation and heartburn.

Raw Only Before Four

Raw foods are highly nutritious but they are also more difficult to digest. In their uncooked forms, they take longer for your body to absorb. If you eat raw food in the evening and then go to sleep, the chances are that these foods will not be digested properly and will hang around in the gut while you slumber. Far from being refreshed, your stomach wakes up to a new job—sorting out last night's dinner. By all means eat raw foods earlier in the day but make sure your body has enough time to deal with them before you go to bed.

5. HOW MUCH TO EAT

Most of us eat too much—more than we need, more than our bodies are designed to cope with and more than our bodies need nutritionally. If your diet is varied enough to include a complete spectrum of vitamins, minerals and amino acids then we don't actually have to eat that much. Yet we do.

This is especially true of products like meat. The definition of "too much" is different for different people, which is why in Mayr therapy treatment plans are always personalized.

Given the strong likelihood that your diet may have been imbalanced for many years towards acid foods, we suggest eating more alkaline foods to compensate—a ratio of 4:1 (alkaline:acid) for a few weeks to really have an effect during the cleanse.

Our stomachs can take up to four hours to process a meal, we need to leave enough time until we eat again. It's not wise to dump fresh food on top of nearly digested food. The stomach needs to deal with one load at a time and customize its acidity accordingly.

Drink water, vegetable tea or herbal tea between meals, but avoid liquids while you are eating.

Portion Control Made Easy

If you fill your stomach with too much food, you will stretch and overwhelm it. We tend to eat meals that are two, three or sometimes four times larger than our stomachs. That's not how we are designed.

If you do this, your body has to pump more and more energy into digesting the unusually large load. This leads to exhaustion of your body's systems, leaving you physically and mentally lacking in energy. Overeating is also wasteful and inefficient—your body can only absorb so many nutrients before your food is excreted. If you eat too much, a lot of the food will just be turned to waste.

Changing portion size is an easy way to reduce your intake. Sometimes in treatments we recommend literally using smaller plates to eat off of, or a teaspoon rather than a tablespoon to give ourselves a visual explanation of what we are trying to achieve. Make every mouthful count and enjoy eating.

6. STAY HYDRATED

Water is one of the most important aspects of an alkaline diet. It helps clean the body and keeps us hydrated. This obviously requires us to start drinking it early in the morning and also develop a taste and respect for it. Drinking water helps circulate nutrients around the body and flushes out toxins. Keeping hydrated is also particularly good for the skin. Given how important it is, it is worth taking more seriously.

The more liquid you can consume, the more it will help to cleanse the body. You should drink at least half a gallon of water a day (if you weigh around 150 pounds, more if you are heavier). Plain water is the best option; however, liquids easily combine, so tisanes, herbal teas and vegetable teas can contribute to your intake.

However, drinking while eating is not good because it dilutes your valuable saliva and stomach acid. Drink half an hour before or after meals. If you have water at the table, the temptation is to wash your food down your throat. Not only will that dilute the saliva and deprive your stomach of an important stimulus, but it also creates a distraction to the main event, digesting food. Water is valuable but not at the same time as food. There is drinking time and there is eating time.

A Note on Alkaline Water

Alkaline, or ionized, water is water that has a pH reading above 7. Like alkaline foods, alkaline water can be used to counteract the effects of an over-acidic diet. Water can be alkalized by using mechanized ionizers and distillers, but two much simpler methods to improve your water's alkalinity are to either add a little baking soda or squeeze a few drops of lemon or lime into a warm glass of water. Both lemon and lime, though acidic, are alkaline-forming.

THE WORLD OF WATER

Pure Water

Pure water is clean, filtered water free from bacteria. It is not mineral-rich and serves to cleanse the body, rather than enrich it. It should have a pH value of 7 and, as such, is neutral. All water may seem neutral in pH but this is not the case, as you will read.

Bottled and Mineral Water

Good minerals in water are especially valuable because we digest them more easily when we drink them rather than eat them. Bottled mineral waters vary widely between very alkaline and mildly alkaline. Oftentimes the pH of bottled mineral water will be listed on the label, but you can easily check for yourself with a pH strip.

Popular brands vary a lot in their levels of minerality. Bicarbonates are alkalizing, so together with dissolved solids such as calcium and magnesium they can create a beneficial effect that will restore nutrients directly to the bone structures that the body may have used in fighting off acid attacks.

In the morning, absorbing fewer minerals is better because you really just want to flush the system. However, in the afternoon, mineral water is an ideal way of delivering minerals to your body.

Distilled Water

Distilled water, while exceptionally pure and free of impurities, is known as "dead water," because it has lost the ability to polarize light and, thus, it has no energetic value for the cells.

Tap Water

Tap water is more likely to be acidic than alkaline, and while that is not a significant issue because the acidity is low, you can nevertheless alkalize it. However, be aware that tap water often contains unwanted chemicals (e.g. chlorine, fluoride, pesticides, etc.) or heavy metals (e.g. aluminum, lead, etc.) so water filtration is advised.

7. EXERCISE REGULARLY

Exercise aids weight loss, strengthens muscles (which support your skeletal system), improves blood flow and stimulates the brain to produce dopamine—a hormone known to lift mood.

The stronger you are physically, the better you support your digestive system. For instance, core fitness supports the intestinal system. Regular exercise does not have to be strenuous to be beneficial. Walking is a natural motion; running long distances perhaps less so. Body movements that shift your frame, your stomach and your chest are a part of keeping supple and toned. You should aim for a minimum of thirty minutes of deliberate cardio exercise every day—walk to work, bike or take the stairs instead of the elevator. Some simple stretching exercises are good, too. We recommend using walking sticks—the ones used for Alpine walking—because they open up the chest, involve the top half of the torso and stop you from hunching.

Be Gentle with Your Body

Be realistic and mindful of your current health status. Exercise in moderation. This not a competition; it is about you and making you feel better. Excessive exercise can be acid-forming. Short, sharp bursts of exercise are fine occasionally if you enjoy them but they are not strictly necessary. It is a regular routine of steady body movement that will deliver the important results. Routine is the key word here, but avoid repetition. Vary the types of exercise you do and the parts of your body that you focus on.

Find Your Naturally Healthy Shape

The point of exercise is to keep our bodies functioning through their natural easy rhythms that support our natural shape. When we become sedentary the very shapes of our bodies change and our internal organs can struggle to operate freely under the pressure. If we drive too much we are hunched over the steering wheel. Bending over a keyboard is like locking yourself into a single mold. We need to break that and stretch back into place. Book dance classes, if necessary.

8. CLEANSE YOUR SYSTEM

Franz Xaver Mayr worked for many years at the Carlsbad spa. There he learned the therapeutic value of the highly mineralized Carlsbad waters. Today at the Original F.X. Mayr & More Health Center we use Epsom salts as a purgative: one level tablespoon to one cup of warm water that is to be drunk in the morning on an empty stomach. It is important to note that though we do not recommend you do this intestinal cleanse at home without supervision.

The scientific name for Epsom salt is magnesium sulphate, and it is the same highly mineralized salt that is used in agriculture to put magnesium (an essential element of the chlorophyll molecule found in plants) back into the soil.

The effect is to put internal pressure on the intestinal tract and to stimulate the liver and the gall bladder, our two main defoliating agents, by squeezing the bile out of the gall bladder, which makes the liver produce new bile. This cleans out any long-standing toxins that may have built up over time and encourages the intestine to start to do the job that it may have been impaired in doing.

Give Your Stomach a Rest

Allowing your body time to recuperate is an important part of Mayr therapy, and the first week of the Alkaline Cure is designed to give your digestive system a rest. Rest for the stomach means reducing the amount you eat, eating nutritionally beneficial foods and simplifying the combinations of foods so they are easy to ingest. Resting the stomach may also involve simple fasting where you consume only tea or water so as not to stress the stomach.

After the stomach has rested, you can begin to introduce varying levels of meals, where different ingredients and recipes are introduced at different stages.

9. ENRICH YOUR SURROUNDINGS

At the health center we enjoy the wonderful forest and mountains around us. The lake that Mayr & More sits on, Lake Wörthersee, is unusual in that it is a full-working recreational lake but the waters are still clean enough to drink. We are fortunate to have hot summers and snowy winters so we can enjoy the seasons and the fresh air. At times we may take our environment for granted, but not everyone is so lucky.

How we live is also a reminder of how we are setting out to cleanse and improve our inner health. A few visible, everyday symbols are worth acquiring: candles that offer a natural light; calming music that is something to look forward to; a new water jug and glass. Simple things that help mark your progress.

Create a Healthy Home Environment

Your home environment has a significant impact on your health and well-being. Even if you live in an inner-city apartment, making a few changes to your home can bring enormous benefits:

* Buy some fresh flowers and plants for each room. They remind us of nature, remove toxins from the air and produce oxygen. According to researchers at Kansas State University, adding plants to hospital rooms was shown to speed recovery rates of surgical patients.

* Open the windows to improve air flow.

* Play pleasurable music—either to energize or relax you.

* Turn off computers and electrical devices in the bedrooms when not in use, but especially when sleeping at night. Appliance lights can stimulate your senses and prevent full, deep sleep. Some also believe that overexposure to the radiation from electrical devices can impact your health.

10. FIND YOUR RHYTHM

Life is rhythms and cycles. Day. Night. Summer. Winter. Our bodies are a part of these natural cycles. Sometimes we have to remind ourselves that these changes are good—even a harsh winter after summer purges the ground as well as our souls. We work hard, we rest, we sleep, we are renewed and we start again. These rhythms and cycles are essential to our well-being. Not following these natural cycles would be turning ourselves into mechanical clockwork machines.

We are not machines but we sometimes drive ourselves like we are. Of course it is admirable to work long hours and to push ourselves and to achieve. But once we have achieved what we set out to do, we must allow our bodies time to recuperate. We need to find the off switch and turn off the engine. It is not lazy to break off and take time out. It is necessary.

Settle and Restore

If you eat on the run, if you squeeze meals between other activities, you are overruling your body's natural instinct to settle and restore. You are stressing it. If necessary we have to reinvent these restorative rhythms and create breaks through the day.

When you go on vacation you can immediately feel the benefit of change. Your ordinary world shrinks and you don't care so much about the things that seemed so important last week. You get some sunshine and you feel better. The body also feels better and is better able to release acids naturally in a hot and sunny climate. In winter it tends to want to cling on to them in case it might need them. During the cold months it is okay to find energy in hot foods like porridge, but in the summer your body wants salads and fruits. Follow its seasonal instincts.

Equally, if you are one of those people who does not like to eat breakfast early in the morning, that is fine—eat a bit later when you are ready. Adjust your routine to suit you. If you are happy on two meals a day, that is fine. If you feel you need four meals, that's okay—just make them smaller. Take control of your routine and your body will be grateful.

Your Body's Thermostat

Your body regulates its own temperature for
different times of the day. At night, it cools internally
for sleep, which is why hot baths help muscles relax—a hot
external environment causes the body to cool down inside.
For daily activity the body needs to be warmer, which is
why a cool shower raises your internal temperature and
primes the body for the day ahead.

Rhythm and Routine

Routines break the day and will give you back a sense of purpose.
Have a glass of warm water when you wake up. Start the day with
a skinbrush and morning shower. Open the windows and try some
stretching. Go for a short walk to breathe the air outside and then
have breakfast.

Rest and Recuperation

With the increasing speed and intensity of modern living, rest is as
important as work—even a nap in the afternoon can be a good thing.
You must realize that you cannot keep doing everything all the time.
Try to interrupt your working routine every ninety minutes or so.
Ideally, you should operate on ninety-minute cycles—seventy-five
minutes of concentration and fifteen minutes of rest and recuperation.
This time should be a deliberate intervention. Open a window or
go for a stroll. And be sure to make time for lunch—thirty minutes
eating time at least. Remember to mix up your restorative activities.
Create a water break in the afternoon. If you get tired later in the day
it may well be due to the foods you ate at lunch that were probably
too quickly eaten. If you're in a hurry, don't gulp down food. It's much
better for you to wait until you have more time to eat.

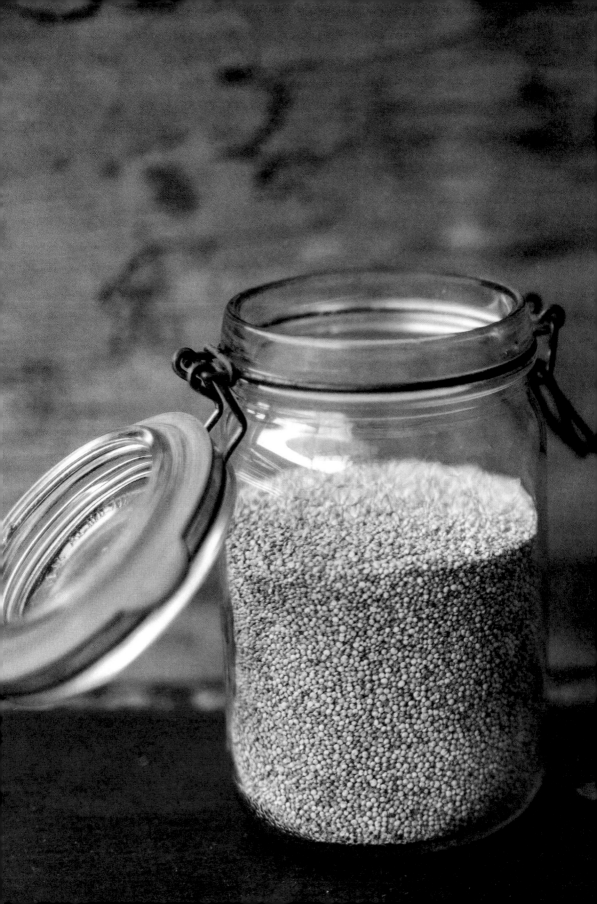

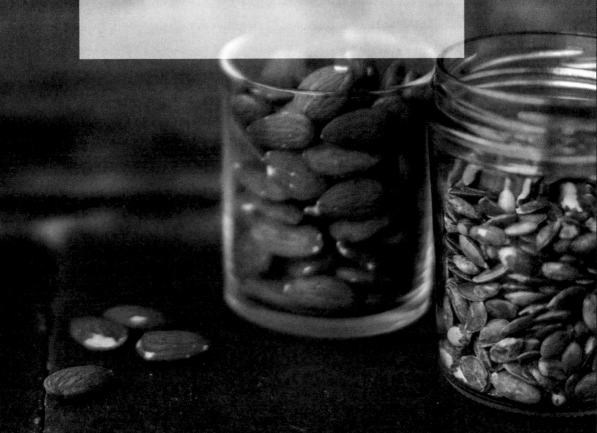

4

Preparing To Go Alkaline

An Alkaline Way of Life
Acid Food Groups
Alkaline Food Groups
20 Alkaline Superfoods
The Alkaline Kitchen

AN ALKALINE WAY OF LIFE

Before starting the Alkaline Cure, it's important to understand the food around you and its impact on your body. By outlining the associated benefits and harmful effects of alkaline and acidic foods, we hope that you will be able to shop and fill your pantry more conscientiously. Once you've set up your alkaline kitchen and are familiar with the foods, tools and cooking methods, you can then start on the quick and easy road to an alkaline way of life.

HOW THE BODY USES FOOD

Food contains nutrients that provide our body with energy and help control growth. There are six main groups of nutrients that the body needs: water, carbohydrates, protein, fats, minerals and vitamins.

Water: The Holy Grail of Health

We can live without the other five nutrients for weeks, but we can only survive a few days without water. It forms the basis of our blood, digestive juices, urine and perspiration. Water's functions include regulating body temperature through sweating, maintaining the health and integrity cells, lubricating joints, carrying nutrients and oxygen to cells and moisturizing skin to maintain its texture and appearance.

Carbohydrates: Fast and Slow Release Energy

Your body uses carbohydrates to make glucose for energy. You find carbohydrates in fruit, vegetables, grains, milk and any food that contains sugar. There are three types of carbohydrates—sugar, starch and fiber—split into two categories, simple and complex. Sugar is simple, meaning your body metabolizes it straight away for energy.

Starch and fiber are complex carbohydrates. Starch-rich foods, such as beans and grains, provide slow-release energy, since your body has to break the starch down into sugar before it can use it. Fiber serves to accelerate the movement of food through the system and affects how nutrients are absorbed.

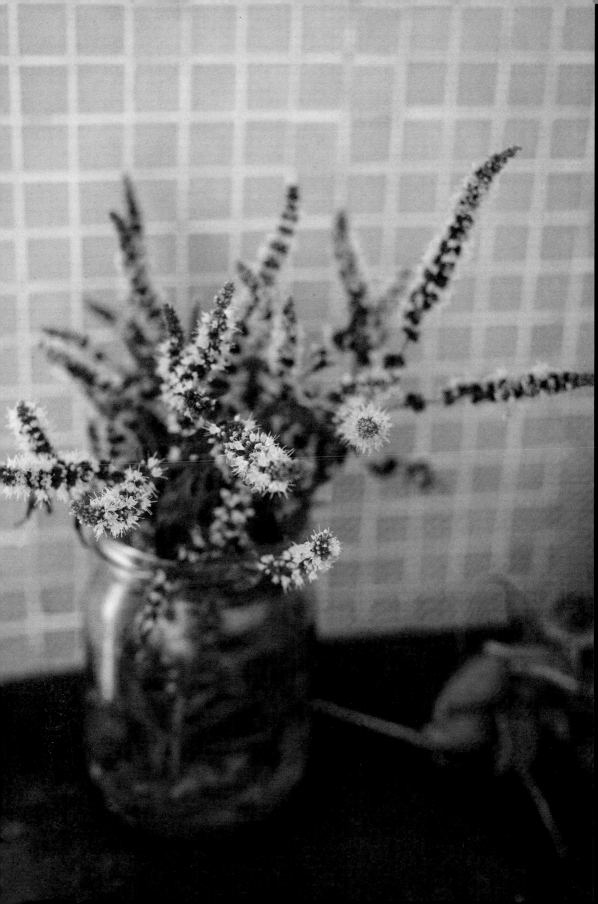

Protein: The Building Blocks of DNA

All foods contain protein but in varying amounts. Protein is made up of chains of amino acids—the building blocks of DNA. Your body needs nine essential amino acids from your diet since it cannot synthesize these for itself. A complete protein is a single food source that contains the nine amino acids in the correct proportions. There are not many complete protein foods, which is why you need to eat a varied diet to gain all the essential amino acids.

Fats and Oils: The Good, the Bad and the Ugly

Fats are essential for energy, proper brain and nerve function, healthy skin and transporting the fat-soluble vitamins A, D, E and K.

There are various categories, with unsaturated being the healthiest, followed by the unhealthier saturated and finally the unhealthiest—trans. Unsaturated fats are mostly found in plant-based foods such as nuts, seeds, vegetable oils and cold-water fish, as well as olive oil, rapeseed oil, peanuts and avocados. Saturated fats are found mostly in animal products—meat, cheese, milk, butter and eggs. Trans fats can be natural or artificial but are mostly created through hydrogenation, a process that is used in the production of fast foods, fried foods and commercial baked products.

Minerals: Strong Bones and Healthy Blood

Minerals are inorganic nutrients that perform a variety of functions. Calcium and magnesium, for example, are important for remineralizing bones and teeth. Iron is a component of hemoglobin, which carries oxygen in red blood cells. The best mineral and vitamin sources include vegetables, fruits and animal products.

Vitamins: The Full Spectrum

Our bodies need a variety of vitamins to stay healthy. Vitamin A helps skin and hair grow. Vitamin C helps fight infections. Vitamin D, synthesized by the skin using sunlight, aids teeth and bone growth.

ACID FOOD GROUPS

The foods below are divided by the strength of their acidity.
Remember rather than cutting all acid foods out entirely, we advise
that you reduce your acid food consumption and compensate by
introducing more alkaline foods into your diet.

Strongly Acid-forming Foods

Animal protein: pork, fish, chicken, lamb, beef

*

Aged dairy products: matured cheese

*

Refined oils and fats: margarine, corn oil

*

Industrially processed products, canned foods

*

Foods containing refined sugar and
flour: preserves, soda, cakes, candy, white bread

*

Coffee, alcohol

Mildly Acid-forming Foods

Vegetable protein: chickpeas, beans, lentils

*

Fresh dairy products: fresh cheese

*

Nuts: cashews, peanuts, pistachios

ACID-FORMING FOODS

Animal Protein and Fish

When we digest foods with sulfur-containing amino acids, like animal proteins, our bodies produce sulfuric acid as a metabolic by-product. So all meat is acidic, almost by definition, although prime cuts tend to be less acidic than fattier parts and fresh meats less acidic than processed meats, which pick up a lot of additives and preservatives. For these reasons we advise that you eat meat only every other day.

Fish is another source of protein that is not alkaline but can offer nutritional benefits such as omega-3 fats and complements alkaline vegetables, such as leeks, spinach, potatoes and red peppers—so we could term fish "alkaline friendly" for that reason.

Milk and Dairy

Fresh milk and fresh cheese can feature in an alkaline diet, although they are slightly acidic as they consist primarily of animal protein and fat. F.X. Mayr was a great advocate for milk as a nutritious food but his milk was unpasteurized and from organic farms near the health center. Over the years pasteurization has become standard but the process of heating depletes milk of much of its nutritional value. With cheese, goat's milk cheese is easier to digest and better for those with allergies than cow's milk cheese.

A Note on Curd Cheese

Curd cheese is similar to quark and cottage cheese. It is a by-product of souring milk with rennet or lemon to separate curds and whey. If you cannot find it locally, then you can drain cottage cheese through muslin and then mash it removing the liquid. As an alternative you can also use thick probiotic yogurt.

Vegetable Protein
Many vegetable proteins are mildly acidic such as chickpeas, lentils, some soy products and certain types of beans, but they have the advantage of not containing cholesterol like animal proteins.

Bread
The yeast in bread tends to encourage an acidic atmosphere in your body and is directly implicated as a source of candida. By avoiding yeast products you may find yourself less bloated. Gluten reactions from wheat and rye tend to be more noticeable as we age, so focus on flatbreads, crispbreads or any breads that are made without yeast.

Refined Oils and Fats
Refined oils and fats tend to be higher in saturated and trans fats, the former more dangerous than the latter. Both raise bad cholesterol, increasing the risk of heart disease, but trans fats also lower good cholesterol and therefore can be more damaging.

Refined Sugar
There is enough natural sugar in our diet without supplementing it. While it's best to avoid adding sugar to food, if you need it, there are natural alternatives such as stevia, which is sweeter than cane sugar.

It's important to note that the sugar in fruit is better than sugar on its own or in processed food since fruit contains fiber, which slows sugar's metabolic rate and prevents an insulin spike.

Caffeine and Alcohol
Caffeine is among the most acidic foods you can consume. The occasional freshly ground coffee is fine; however, daily consumption is known to leach minerals from bones to buffer the acidity caused by the caffeine.

Alcohol sits on the acid throne alongside caffeine. Try to avoid drinking alcohol in general, but if you do, favor quality as often as possible, such as additive- and preservative-free organic beers.

ALKALINE FOOD GROUPS

Nearly all vegetables, herbs, root spices (such as garlic and ginger), many fruits (provided they are ripe) and cold-pressed oils are alkaline. Some people are sensitive to certain vegetables, and if you feel they are not doing you any good then simply avoid them.

Alkaline-forming Foods

Vegetables: broccoli, cabbage, spinach, kale,
salad leaves, potatoes, sweet potatoes, sprouts, beets,
cucumber

*

Ripe fruits: bananas, watermelon, papaya, mango

*

New and ancient grains: amaranth, quinoa,
rye, buckwheat

*

Fresh, aromatic herbs: basil, rosemary, thyme

*

Nuts: almonds

*

High-quality, cold-pressed "virgin"
vegetable, nut and seed oils: flaxseed oil, olive oil,
pumpkin seed oil, hempseed oil

*

Pure and mineral water, herbal teas,
vegetable tea

ALKALINE-FORMING FOODS

Vegetables have always been a crucial part of an alkaline diet. Not only are they nutritional powerhouses, but vegetables have even become fashionable in high-class cooking. In Paris, Alain Passard has three Michelin stars for his restaurant L'Arpège where each day one menu is dedicated to the produce from his garden. He offers dishes such as celery risotto with herb emulsion, celeriac mousseline with turnips and lemon, and root vegetables with couscous, Argan oil and celery emulsion—all alkaline in extremis.

An alkaline diet is a prescription for a healthier lifestyle and also healthier agriculture. Our taste buds instinctively prefer fresh and locally grown—or, even better, homegrown—vegetables because their nutritional value diminishes if they are left to linger in the back of a truck, on a supermarket shelf or, worse, in a warehouse.

It is never a question of either-or with vegetables. Cooking two, three or even four kinds of vegetables together brings color and vitality to the plate as well as a more complete nutritional spectrum—color on the plate is always good.

Leafy Green Vegetables

Green and leafy vegetables such as broccoli, sprouts, cabbage and spinach are more than just backdrops on the plate. They are high in vitamin A—essential for healthy skin, hair and nails—and vitamin C, a potent antioxidant. Kale and other leafy greens are a good source of iron and calcium. These veggies are versatile in cooking, adding fresh and interesting flavors to dishes. The water in which a cauliflower is steamed also makes excellent stock for an alkaline vegetable tea. The leaves around a cauliflower are nutritious and tasty.

Salad leaves are more than just garnish, they're a valuable first course and a way of incorporating vegetable oil dressings (such as pumpkin oil, virgin olive oil and flaxseed oil), seeds, small fruits (such as cranberries and pomegranate seeds), and a generous handful of fresh herbs. All salad leaves are alkaline. Lettuce is surprisingly nutritious: two cups of romaine lettuce will give you more than enough vitamin A and K for the day. Iceberg is not quite as nutritious but still contains vitamin B, potassium, manganese, iron, calcium and phosphorous. It

A Note on Antioxidants

Antioxidants are nutrients and enzymes that help
fight the damaging effects of free radicals by neutralizing
them. Free radicals are highly reactive chemicals that
damage our cells and are said to cause cancer. Alkalizing
foods, such as strawberries, prunes, kale and spinach, are
packed with antioxidants including beta-carotene,
lycopene, and vitamins A, C and E.

also contains a fair amount of copper and zinc. The zesty arugula is a
rich food in terms of minerals and vitamins. Any alkaline lunch can
start with a good salad.

Sprouts

One of the most nutritious of all vegetables are sprouting seedlets,
of which alfalfa is one of the most commonly found. Other pulses can
be sprouted as well. Sprouting boosts nutritional value, and sprouts are
often easier for the body to digest. Sprouting is a fun and easy kitchen
activity that bears valuable results.

Roots and Tubers

Roots and tubers provide the framework for an alkaline diet—not just
potato but beet, carrot, celeriac, parsnips, radish, swede and turnip are
all planks and girders of an alkaline meal. Steamed, mashed, baked,
they submit happily to nearly every culinary innovation. Some, such as
carrot and celeriac, are also famously good just grated into their own
raw salad—the former with a few currants and an orange dressing, the
latter with a flaxseed mayonnaise.

Other Vegetables

All squashes are alkaline alongside zucchini, cucumber and pumpkin.
The stem and stalk vegetables—such as artichoke, asparagus, celery

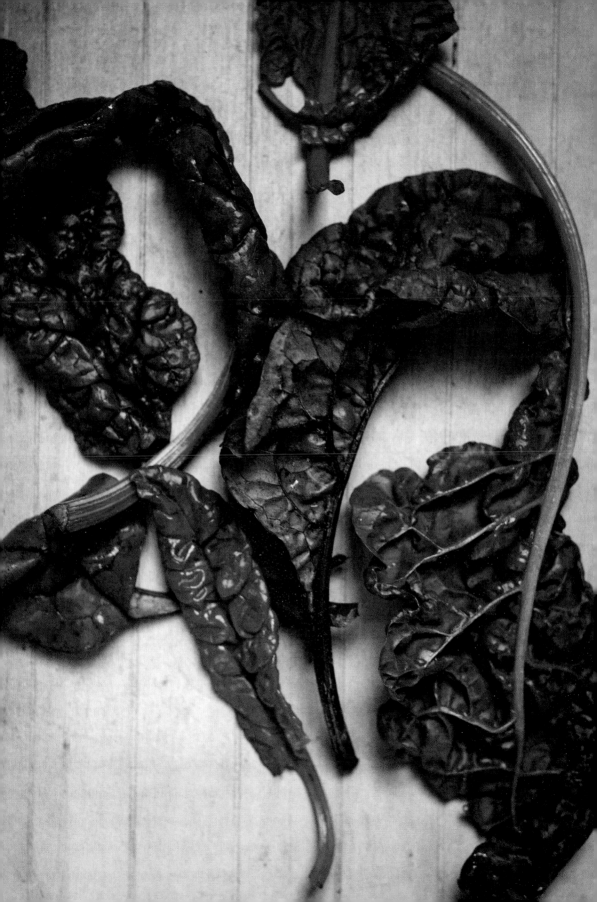

and fennel—again are all alkaline and packed with minerals, vitamins, and fiber. A meal comprised of one vegetable from each of the above sections would be a feast indeed and nearly all can be liquidized into purees and spreads to bring other dimensions into your eating.

We tend to take onions and leeks for granted but both are the base of many regional cuisines around the world and are an easy way to slip some fresh alkalizing vitamins into your cooking.

FRUIT

The problem with fruit is that, very often, it is not ripe. If fruit has not had enough time to ripen naturally—or has been chemically ripened in storage—then it simply does not have the same nutritional values that we are expecting.

A strawberry rushed around the globe to decorate a supermarket shelf will not have the same value as a strawberry fresh picked from a garden in the ideal season. Tomatoes, too, are classified as a fruit and need to be very ripe for maximum nutritional benefit. As bananas ripen, indicated by brown spots, the starch starts to turn to sugar which provides excellent fast-acting energy for our cells.

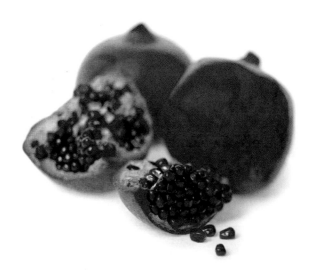

Melons are a wonderful alkaline fruit and can be easily digested because they are mostly water. As such, the body absorbs their nutrients quickly and easily. Watermelon is one of the most alkaline of all fruits.

Dried Fruit

Drying fruits can be an effective way of preserving the alkalinity, especially in ripe fruits, provided they have not been dipped in a solution of ascorbic acid, citric acid, sodium metabisulfite or sugar, which can all undermine the fruit's alkalinity. Read the labels. Properly and naturally dried fruits such as currants, apricots, mangoes, plums and bananas can be welcome alkaline additions to snacks, breakfasts and salads. The low temperatures of drying in the oven or in a specialist food dehydrator help retain nutrients that cooking might otherwise destroy.

Dried fruit can form an important source of fiber, potassium, vitamins and minerals—for example, apricots and peaches contain vitamin A for skin support, figs contain calcium for bones and plums contain vitamin K, which can help ease constipation and promote healthy bone development.

If you are drying fruit at home then use lemon to preserve, which underlines the alkalizing effect and prevents discoloration. Drying can be a lengthy process: thin apple slices will take about six hours in an oven at 140°F (60°C) and peach halves may take up to thirty-six hours.

GRAINS

Grains are incredibly versatile and nutritious. They have been cultivated and used in various forms for much of human history. But the most popular grain, wheat, is now so widely cultivated, modified and processed that by the time it turns up in supermarkets as bagels and sliced white bread, it has often lost most of its nutritional value.

Commercially, wheat tends to top everything else in terms of being fast-growing, high-yielding and hardier than other crops. But it is only when we look at the health benefits of other grains that we can see how other crops offer more nutritional depth and benefits.

A Note on Gluten

Awareness of gluten intolerance has increased in
recent years. At the health center we test every patient who
comes through. Sometimes, eating less gluten is enough to
avoid an allergic reaction, but if you have a gluten allergy
you may have to stick to eating gluten-free grains, such as
millet, or pseudocereals, such as amaranth,
quinoa and buckwheat.

A World of Grains

When we look to the traditional foods of other cultures, we can see
the wide variety of nutritious grains available. Rye contains more
amino acids, fiber and vitamin E than wheat, and it is also has a lower
gluten content. Amaranth and quinoa are high in fiber as well as the
essential amino acid lysine, which helps build body muscle and tissue
and boosts the nutritional impact of the protein sources it is paired
with. Buckwheat is also a source of lysine, and buckwheat noodles—
used as soba noodles in Japan—are a healthy alternative to white pasta.

Amaranth, quinoa and buckwheat, though they can be used and
eaten like other cereals, are actually pseudocereals. True cereals, like
wheat, oats and rice, are derived from grasses, while pseudocereals are
derived from other kinds of plants. Pseudocereals often have a more
complex nutritional profile and do not contain gluten.

Mixing different grains is, in itself, a good diet practice because each
has its own attributes and cocktail of amino acids. And adding healthy
grains to traditional breakfast dishes such as porridge and granola is an
easy way to gain more nutritional benefits from those meals.

THE POWER OF HERBS AND SPICES

Herbs and spices are as universally alkaline as meat is universally acid. They also bring other benefits in terms of minerals and vitamins. The aim is to bring them into our diet more readily so they can start to play a more fundamental role.

Herbs

Parsley is a simple, versatile herb; use it generously. It is rich in antioxidants, potassium, calcium, manganese, iron and magnesium. There are more than thirty varieties, all of which taste markedly different. At one extreme, we have the tightly furled, curly variety and, at the other, the fragrant flat leaf.

Every sprig has two uses: the stalks help make flavorsome stocks and can be added directly into soups—use string to hold them together so they can be taken out later. The leaves can go in at the end of the cooking to add some color and freshness.

Other herbs such as basil, rosemary, thyme, sage, marjoram and chervil all make wonderful additions to meals and bring with them many health benefits as well. These small but potent leaves are packed with everything from antioxidants, potassium, iron and calcium to manganese, magnesium and selenium. Plus they provide the body with B-complex vitamins, beta-carotene, folic acid and vitamins A, K, E and C.

Consequently, they have health benefits to suit their nutritional content. These herbs are known to fight cancer, boost brain function, aid digestion, increase circulation and have anti-inflammatory and antiviral properties.

Root Herbs

Garlic and ginger are some of the more potent members of the root family. Ginger makes a potent tea in itself. More radical, and often recommended for candida, is garlic tea—four peeled and crushed cloves steeped for twenty minutes in four cups of hot water with a grating of ginger and a few drops of lemon. Horseradish has been used for centuries to treat a variety of ailments, from urinary tract infections

A Note on Candida

Candida, a type of yeast, is the most common cause
of fungal infection in humans, and it thrives in acidic
environments. When candida levels get out of control,
they can cause a host of health problems, including yeast
infections, bloating and severe allergic reactions. The best
way to treat candida is by healing the gut: eliminating sugar,
fermented foods and alcohol (all of which candida feeds
off of), reducing carbohydrate intake and eating foods that
fight candida, such as garlic, ginger and parsley.

curd, or just a few strings off a grater can dramatically change the taste
of a dish. It goes especially well with beets.

Seeds and Spices
Although small, seeds deliver a disproportionately high nutritional
value into the diet. Seeds need to be freshly ground and will not
keep for more than a few hours. Flaxseed, sunflower seeds, pine nuts,
pumpkin seeds, sesame seeds and wheat germ are all good alkaline
companions to sprinkle on salads or on porridge. Seeds can also be
sprouted, much like alfalfa.

Spices derive from seeds. A grinder or a pestle and mortar can
create new spice mixes—such as coriander and fennel seeds—and be
scattered on cooked dishes. Or put spices in a pepper mill on the table
for everyone else to help themselves. Spices are a quick way to spike
your food, both taste-wise and nutritionally.

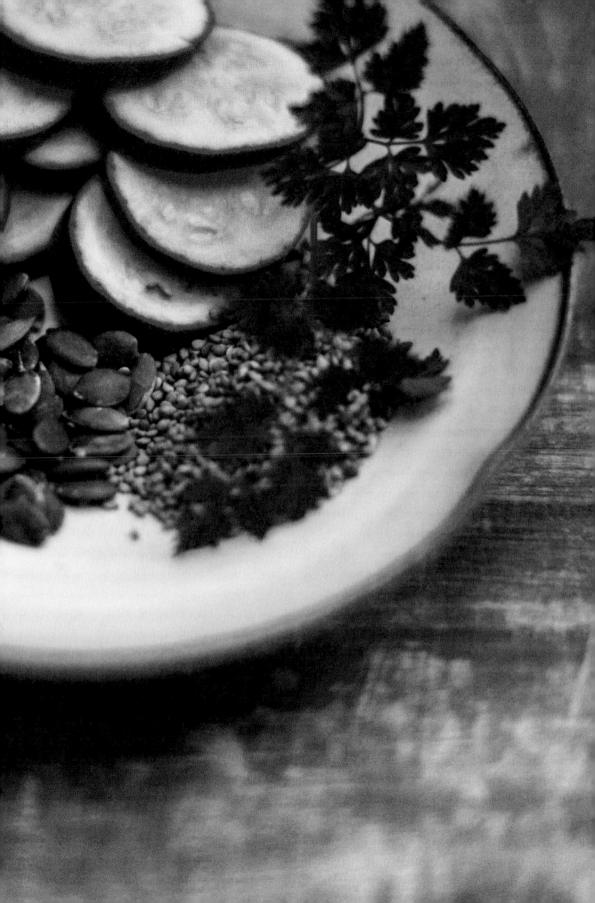

20 ALKALINE SUPERFOODS

All alkaline foods have incredible health benefits that will contribute to your overall health. Nevertheless, these twenty alkaline superfoods are our choices for the most beneficial alkaline ingredients.

Avocado
This creamy, highly alkaline fruit provides nearly twenty essential nutrients, including fiber, potassium, vitamin E and B vitamins.

Pumpkin
Members of the pumpkin and squash family contain high levels of essential omegas-3 and -6 fats. They are also high in vitamin A, vitamin C and a number of B vitamins. Roast their seeds for a high-protein snack, and use pumpkin oil in salads.

Potato
Rich in healthy carbohydrates, potatoes are a great source of alkalinity. Potatoes bind acids in the stomach—this alkaline effect benefits the entire body. Their nutritional profile includes vitamin C, iron, magnesium and potassium.

Amaranth
These seeds are tan or light brown and very small like poppy seeds. They are notably high in the amino acid lysine, which is not true of other grains, and fiber. Just six ounces supply the equivalent of all the protein one might need in a day. It can be toasted, treated like popcorn, scattered on salads or used as a thickener for soups or as a breakfast porridge base.

Celery

Long filled with peanut butter as the staple of children's birthday parties, celery is a valuable source of alkaline nutrition. It is particularly at home in soups and chopped over salads. It contains calcium and niacin, which means it helps with digestion and lowers blood pressure.

Celeriac

Related to celery, celeriac is a root vegetable with an impressive number of vitamins, minerals and benefits. It contains B vitamins, vitamin C and vitamin K, as well as phosphorous, iron, calcium, magnesium and antioxidants. The aniseed-tasting celeriac can be grated in salads, steamed, mashed and made into gratins.

Kale

Of all the healthy, leafy brassicas, kale is perhaps the most beneficial, boasting a long list of vitamins and minerals—especially calcium, iron, magnesium and phosphorus. Despite having such a strong flavor, kale can easily be balanced with other foods to create nutritious and delicious salads, smoothies and stews.

Almonds

Not technically a true nut, the seed of the almond is what we eat. They are high in protein and calcium, as well as being a source of zinc and vitamin E. Almond flour makes a great baking alternative. Almonds also produce a calming effect and provide essential nutrients for your skin.

Carrot

Carrots are filled with calcium, magnesium, potassium and beta-carotene, which metabolizes into vitamin A and encourages healthy eyesight. Carrots also help cleanse the liver and, therefore, are perfect as part of a cleanse.

Quinoa

Originating in the Andes, quinoa is a versatile, gluten-free seed, or "pseudocereal." It is exceptionally high in calcium as well as being a rich source of fiber, magnesium and iron. It can be prepared as a meal base and then eaten hot or cold, similar to the way one would eat rice. And considering the high protein content, nutritionally, it wins out against its more famous counterpart.

Beet

Beets are as rich in nutrients as they are in color. A great source of folate, beets also contain calcium, vitamin C and potassium, among other nutrients. They have been shown to reduce kidney stones and lower blood pressure and the risk of cardiovascular disease.

Oils

More and more research has highlighted flaxseed oil (also known as linseed oil) as one of the most beneficial oils because it provides a source of omega-3 fatty acids. Also good are cold-pressed olive, hemp, pumpkin and other nut and seed oils, which can bring splendid color as well as nutritional value to your cooking.

Broccoli

This dark leafy-green vegetable of the cabbage family contains high amounts of vitamin C, calcium and dietary fiber. It serves as an antioxidant, antiviral and antibiotic liver stimulant.

Ginger

Traditionally used to combat nausea, ginger root has many other uses both in medicine and in the kitchen. It can also be made into tea or used to make cookies and breads. Ginger is a source of calcium, magnesium, potassium and phosphorous, all of which improve circulation, stimulate the liver and act as an antispasmodic.

Watermelon, Mango and Papaya
Watermelon is a wonderfully refreshing and hydrating fruit. Easily digested due to its high water content, it is high in vitamins C and A, offering anti-inflammatory and antioxidant properties. Mango is a luxurious fruit, delicious on its own or in desserts and salads, and is extremely high in vitamin C and dietary fiber. The exotic papaya with its beautifully colored flesh contains three times your daily vitamin C requirements, providing good immune system and skin support.

Fennel
With its fine leaves and long slender stalks anchored by a nutritious bulb, this alkaline superfood is rich in vitamin C, fiber, potassium and manganese. It has anti-inflammatory and antioxidant properties and helps boost your immune system.

Figs
Rich in B vitamins, vitamin K, potassium, iron, magnesium and omega fatty acids, figs are a sweet way to improve your brain function, prevent cancer, build bones and protect your heart. Figs are also a source of dietary fiber. They can be enjoyed both fresh (when available) as well as dried.

Coconut
All over the world various parts of the coconut are used for various purposes. The water can be drunk as an energizing antioxidant drink, the milk can promote weight maintenance and the oil is a healthier cooking alternative to other cooking oils. Coconuts are high in phosphorous, magnesium and potassium, and when added to various dishes both sweet and savory, can lift the flavor and add sweetness.

THE ALKALINE KITCHEN

You should try to organize your kitchen to make it alkaline-friendly, so that it is easier to work in and you have the essential equipment on hand that will allow you to cook up a healthier lifestyle. You can, of course, cook almost anything in this book with a knife, a pan and a stove top, but some kits and gadgets will make life easier and the cooking more fun.

If you enjoy your cooking, then you will enjoy the eating. The same rules apply. The kitchen should be a calm, therapeutic space. Turning it into a pleasant place to be will make you feel better and that feeling will extend to the dishes you prepare. Food is only one part of the alkaline approach and preparing it has to follow the same principles of calmness and well-being.

Alkaline on a Budget
You may be surprised at how much money you will save by following an alkaline diet. A great deal of the foods we recommend are reasonably inexpensive—especially vegetables, even if you are paying for premium organic produce. You can afford to pay more for herbs and buy bigger quantities. Cold-pressed oils are relatively more expensive than bulk vegetable oils but they are a vital component of the diet, and, again, you are only using small quantities so you can afford to build up a collection of different oils over the weeks. When you are buying meat or fish, try to buy the best cuts with the money you have saved from the rest of your shop.

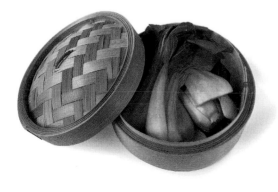

A KITCHEN EQUIPMENT CHECKLIST

Steamer: use a steamer to steam rather than boil vegetables. Chinese-style bamboo steaming baskets are good for stacking and steaming different vegetables at the same time

Soup pan: large casseroles or saucepans are useful for cooking soups and stews

Nonstick pans: with nonstick pans you do not have to use fats and oils for frying

Grater: graters are useful for catching zests of oranges and lemons (check that the fruits have not been waxed) and vegetables for salads or soups

Mandolin: mandolins help to quickly slice vegetables into thin leaves or uniform slices

Coffee grinder: a coffee grinder can mill spices at the last minute. You can also use an old-fashioned pestle and mortar as an alternative

Blender: a simple, handheld stick blender is enough for blending soups, sauces, dips and dressings

Juicer: juicers quickly and easily make vegetable and fruit juices

Knives: a good knife or set of knives that are sharp are always essential items in the kitchen. A small easy-to-handle knife is imperative, as well as a cleaver or larger knife for handling root vegetables

Strainer: use a strainer to easily drain vegetables or strain liquids. You can also use a muslin cloth if you want to get a really clean mix

SHOPPING

Most ingredients in the cure are fairly easy to find, but make sure you choose quality ingredients, because this will make all the difference.

Vegetables and Herbs

Markets are usually the best value for buying vegetables, especially where you can buy single vegetables inexpensively. Fresh and seasonal are best; organic is likely to be better because pesticides are inevitably acidic. Boxed schemes offer convenience and visual affirmation of how many vegetables you should have in your kitchen each week. Herbs can be bought either as the whole plant or in precut bunches.

Fruit

Buy fruit that is properly ripe. Brown spots on bananas or slight softness in fruits such as plums and peaches are obvious signs of ripeness. For melons, you can usually smell the ripeness at the base (though this does not apply to watermelons).

Meat and Fish

Buy the best and the choicest leaner cuts—fillet for beef, loin for pork, cutlets and leg for lamb. Free-range chickens have more texture and flavor and are the more ethical choice.

For fish, fresh is best, always. Try to buy fish on the day you are going to eat it. Frozen is not necessarily a bad option because, often, the fish is frozen at sea after being caught and can therefore be in fairly good condition.

Dairy and Cheese

For the cure we prefer fresh young cheeses—cow's, goat's or sheep's—made from unpasteurized milk to preserve the nutrients.

Grains and Bread

Supermarket breads are increasingly implicated in allergies and gluten intolerance. Opt for crispbreads or bake your own flatbreads without yeast. Grains, such as barley, quinoa and amaranth, can bring new angles to granola and porridges and be substituted in recipes.

ALKALINE PANTRY BASICS

These are non-perishable foods that you will use throughout the fourteen-day Alkaline Cure, so make sure your pantry is stocked with these alkaline staples before starting.

Pantry Basics

Cereals and grains: oats, millet, quinoa, couscous, bulgur
wheat and buckwheat

*

Dried fruit: figs, apricots and prunes

*

Seeds: fennel, coriander, caraway, sunflower,
sesame, pumpkin, flax and cumin

*

Spices: paprika, nutmeg (whole),
rock or sea salt, pepper, curry spice
and cinnamon

*

Oils: olive oil, flaxseed oil, pumpkin oil,
coconut oil and walnut oil

*

Nuts: Almonds, pine nuts, cashews and walnuts

*

Other: baking soda, honey or maple
syrup and crispbread

OILS AND FATS

An alkaline kitchen should have a good range of different oils that can bring new flavors and nutrients to dishes. It is the omega-3, -6 and -9 components that are most valuable here. Omega-6 is found in many different foods including meats, but most of us may have as much as twenty times more compared to the other omegas. Virgin olive oil—also known as cold-pressed—is a familiar standby for omega-9 too, along with other nut and seed oils. Ideally we are looking for a mix of one part omega-3, two parts omega-6 and one part omega-9.

Omega-3 is found mainly in flaxseed oil or cold water fish—it is the omega our grandmothers proudly tried to get us to swallow by the teaspoonful.

These oils are helpful in supporting the enzymes that convert food into energy. Different oils bring different values—a good collection in an alkaline kitchen is inspiring.

The first pressing of an oil, the virgin oil, even if unfiltered will have the most benefits. It is possible sometimes to find first pressings of sunflower and grape seed oils, a state in which they have a useful role in cooking, but general vegetable oils have been denatured and have lost their nutritional value and are deemed acidic.

Maintaining Vitality

Oils are sensitive to light so should be sold in small quantities—for freshness—and in dark-colored glass bottles or tin cans. They are a fresh product and will expire and lose their vitality over time—six months for native oils and maximum a year for other cold-pressed oils.

Pumpkin Oil

Pumpkin oil is a power food, a rich cocktail of nutrients including vitamins A, E, zinc and selenium with an ideal blend of omega-3 and -6 fatty acids. In some Eastern European countries it has earned PDO (Protected Designation of Origin) status and has been part of the diet and herbal therapies in that region for centuries. Its medicinal attributes meant it was often prescribed for irritable bowel syndrome.

Cooking with Oil

The heat of cooking destroys many of the valuable
vitamins and omegas found in cold-pressed oils. For that
reason, add them at the end of the cooking. The same is true
of butter. Many recipes can be grilled rather than
fried. Or use a nonstick pan.

The best oil for cooking because it has the highest
heat resistance is cocnut oil. And it is alkaline—which can
be useful when cooking Asian-style stir-fries, where its
strong flavour tends to complement the flavors
and not overpower them.

Flaxseed Oil

In Eastern Europe flaxseed oil—also called linseed oil—was used as
a dressing for potatoes, and in Indian cooking it is known as *tisi*. It
is rich in omega-3 fats and the flavor can be pronounced. Cultivation
goes back to the Neolithic era, when flax was used to make linen.

Hempseed Oil

Hemp or hempseed oil has a grassy, nutty taste that increases the
darker it is. Not to be confused with the intoxicating hash oil, which is
made from the flowers and leaves of the plant, the oil from the seeds is
of high nutritional value because of its 3:1 ratio of omega-6 to omega-3
essential fatty acids—an ideal concoction. It also contains vitamin D
and high levels of vitamin E.

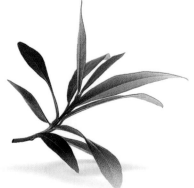

HOW TO COOK

Our cooking times are short because we have learned that overheating food can destroy valuable proteins, enzymes and nutrients. Herbs, in fact, are never cooked at all but only incorporated at the very end of the cooking process. Our restaurant at the health center enjoys a deserved gastronomic reputation and that is because we see no difference between good-tasting food and food that is good for us.

Cooking should be therapeutic and enjoyable, a part of the rhythm of life. It is a good way to create breaks in the day and the evening when you have time to leave other things alone. Like eating, you need to set aside some time to prepare things properly. Cooking should not be a rush, nor a stress. Preparing a good soup can be a pleasurable process—handling raw vegetables and letting them transform into something to look forward to.

Cook vegetables for as short a time as possible. It can be useful to cut vegetables up smaller or even grate them so that they cook quicker.

Stock is often a hurdle for cooks but in the alkaline kitchen it is easy—just reserve the water you used to cook your vegetables and then you will always have a continual supply of fresh stock for poaching or using in soups, which will add extra nutritional goodness. Cooking can and should be a cyclical process.

Breaking the Frying Habit
Poaching or simmering is healthier and can often replace frying. Frying is perhaps more of a habit than a necessity, while deep-fat frying is, by definition, an acidfying process. From an alkaline perspective, most recipes that begin with frying vegetables are off the mark, health-wise. Grilling or broiling is a cleaner option for your meat. Steaming vegetables is better than boiling them. Baking, which essentially is just dry poaching, is equally reliable.

Butter should not be exposed to too much heat when cooking; therefore, a knob on boiled potatoes is fine, especially with a few chopped chives or parsley.

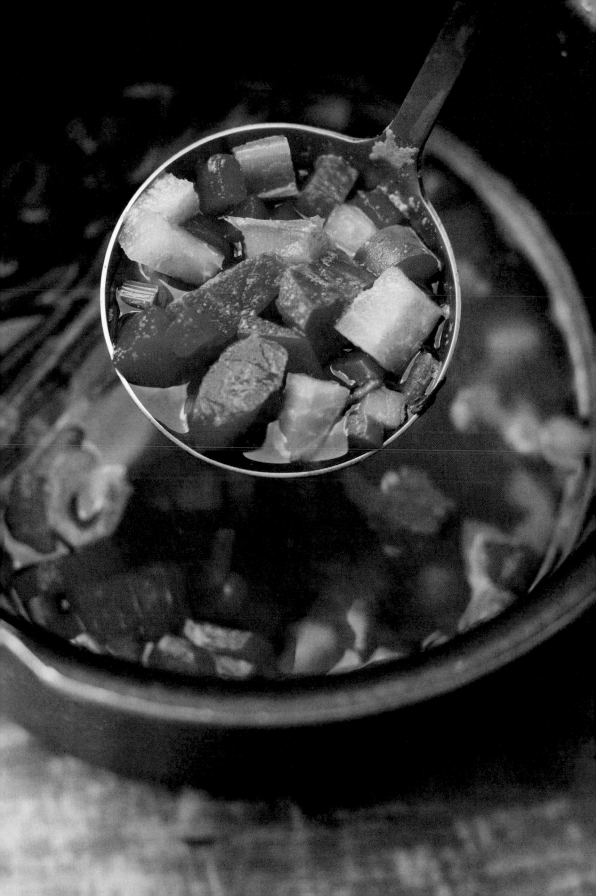

Heaping on the Herbs

Herbs should be used as abundantly as you can, either while cooking or fresh atop a dish. Be extravagant. These are your luxuries; try and enjoy them.

Asian influences offer us many sensible ideas in the kitchen. In Thai cuisine, the holy trinity of seasoning is garlic, ginger and chili—all alkalizing influences. Dishes are garnished not with one or two leaves but handfuls of cilantro and basil.

When cooking with herbs, there are a few things to keep in mind. Remember that basil does not like heat at all, so only add it to dishes at the last minute. Rosemary and thyme are strong tasting and are best used to pass on their aromas in broths and teas. Sage and marjoram are great complementary herbs for poultry and other meats. Chervil adds a delicate flair to dishes.

Store your fresh herbs in jars or cups with the stems in water, like a bouquet of flowers. Change the water regularly. Dried herbs and seeds should be stored in dark, cool places.

Spicing Up Your Life

Herbs and spices can be toasted in a frying pan or dried in the oven quickly and mixed with rock salt to dramatically change the nature of a dish. The typical ingredients of store-bought curry powder are mostly alkaline—coriander seed, cayenne pepper, cumin, garlic, ginger—although you may prefer to make up your own and avoid any preservatives bottled mixes may contain. A coffee grinder doubles up as a spice mill, and if you make too much you can always store it and use it as needed.

Rock and sea salts lend minerals to the diet. Most types of salt taste very different. Much of the sodium impact will depend on the size of the grain or flake, which can also offer textures. A good collection of different salts—like homemade salts with herbs—are fine additions to your kitchen staples.

Whole Foods Versus Purees

Purees for soups and dips offer the fastest, most efficient way of delivering nutritional benefits. They are easier to digest than whole foods, and they can be vehicles for including different flavors, especially herbs, spices and even oils with high omega factors. And for meals later in the day when the body might not have enough time to break down solids, they can play a useful role.

But for most of us, the fiber in foods is also an important aspect of eating and helping teach the body how to digest. Therefore, in principle, whole foods are better. But it is also a question of balance. For example, take an orange. It may take upward of three or four oranges to make a glass of orange juice. That represents quite a nutritional impact compared to eating a few slices of orange. However, the body's digestive system is going to be more comfortable with the orange slices as opposed to the glass of pulped essence with a vitamin content that is sixteen times greater. You may feel like you're getting a whole lot of vitamins, but your body may not agree or be able to benefit from it.

Preserving

Fresh foods are always preferable. The issues with preserving foods from a nutritional point of view are obvious and go further than just concerns about histamine. In extending storage life, fruits, vegetables and other otherwise high-value sources of nutrition inevitably degrade.

Agents used for preserving food—most commonly salt, sugar, vinegar and other additives—are acidic. With very few exceptions, any foods sold in bags, cans, sleeves or other kinds of packaging are very likely to be more acid. Even a microwave dinner that contains ingredients that seem to have an alkaline leaning, when filled with preservatives and packaged, themselves become acidic.

Better to use fresh and cook it yourself. Frozen vegetables without additives, especially for chestnuts, corn and peas, may remain alkaline, but mixes of ingredients for meals are unlikely to sustain their much-needed alkalinity.

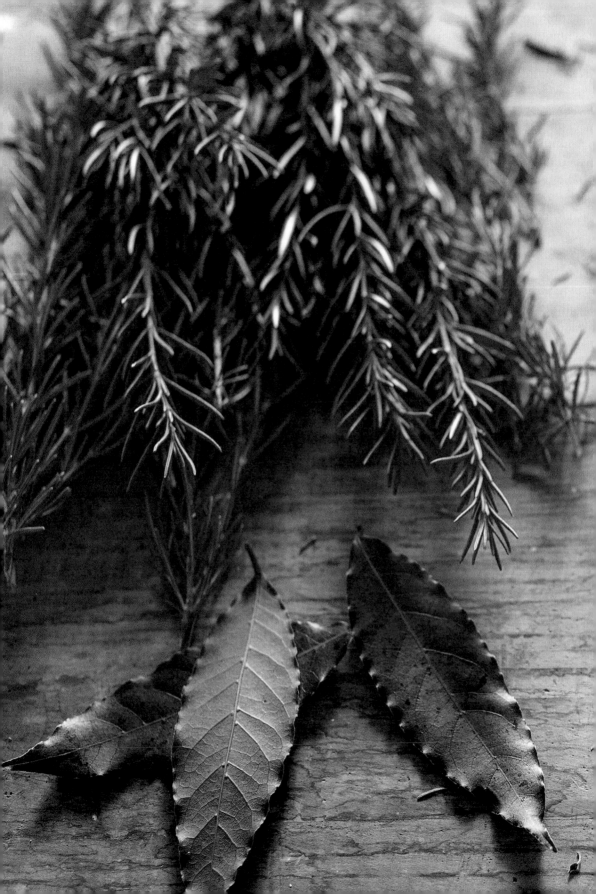

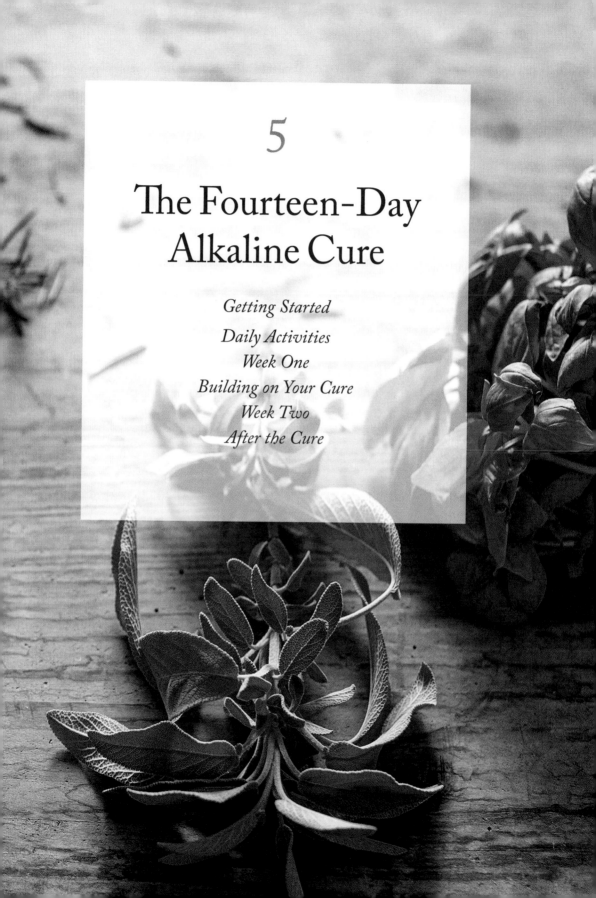

5

The Fourteen-Day Alkaline Cure

Getting Started
Daily Activities
Week One
Building on Your Cure
Week Two
After the Cure

GETTING STARTED

The first week of the Alkaline Cure is designed to cleanse your system. The second week introduces a few more alkaline ingredients and ideas to help make alkaline foods a part of your life.

The best time to start your Alkaline Cure is on a weekend or a day when you are not going to be distracted so you can give yourself enough time to get organized. Keep things simple and straightforward and do what is manageable for your schedule. If you prepare your breakfast the night before, you will have all the elements easily on hand without having to think about it in the morning. Also, if you make up your vegetable tea or soup the night before, it will have time to infuse properly.

Depending on how acidic your body is, you will likely feel some side effects as you go: headaches, fatigue, anxiety, mood changes or cravings. These are good signs, signs that your body is getting rid of toxins. Live with them. They will pass quickly enough. Remember that many of our health problems have built up over several years, and real change may take time. The next fourteen days is a start.

THE WEEK BEFORE YOU START

You might reward yourself with a couple of days of vacation from work to get you up and running. Pencil a date in your calendar and give yourself a few days to get used to the idea. It is also a good idea to adopt a few new changes before starting the Alkaline Cure:

* Cut down on a few small things like coffee, alcohol and carbonated drinks.

* Don't buy any fast food, junk food and packaged food, and clean out your refrigerator and pantry so you are not tempted.

* Cut out sugar, especially refined sugar.

* Start drinking water and get into the habit of drinking half a gallon (two liters) or more a day.

* Get your shopping list together for the first few days so you have everything on hand at home. Do not be tempted to economize on your shopping—the best, freshest produce will create the tastiest, healthiest recipes. Your food portions over the next two weeks will be fairly controlled, so you should be able to afford to be a little extravagant with the quality of your groceries.

* One tip that can help you to start eating less is to use smaller plates. Plate your meals on side plates or in bowls rather than on big dinner plates.

* Start establishing a relaxing new evening routine. For instance, take a walk after dinner and give yourself some personal time to listen to music or read a book. Two hours before bed, take a warm bath.

THE DAY BEFORE YOU START

The day before you start the plan, go shopping and get everything ready in the kitchen. Make your alkaline minestrone (page 140) so you know you have a good, dependable standby waiting for you to enjoy. All of the recipes in the day planner can be found in the next section, listed by category and in order of appearance. For easy reference, a recipe finder can be found at the back of the book. If you cannot get all the ingredients to follow the recipes precisely, it is not crucial; just buy your produce according to the seasons and substitute alkaline vegetables, spices and herbs as you can.

If you are or want to be a vegetarian, substitute the meat-based recipes in the day planner with any of the menu options that are marked with a ❶ in the recipe section.

Since exercise is such an important part of the Alkaline Cure, the evening before you begin, take a gentle stroll outside. For the plan, we have provided you with new exercises to try every day that alternate between cardio, stretching, breathing and core exercises. We have also given beauty and environment suggestions to help you create an alkaline lifestyle. The "In the Kitchen" section of the day planner has suggestions for dishes you can make in the evening for the following day's meals.

DAILY ACTIVITIES

A daily routine is good. While taking the Alkaline
Cure, try to do the following every day:

* **Dry brush your skin:** before your daily bath or shower,
  take a loofah or natural bristle brush and gently dry brush
  your skin. It will eliminate dead skin cells, unblock pores,
  kickstart the lymph system and increase blood circulation.

* **Gargle with flaxseed oil:** an oil mouthwash is an effective
  way of cleaning your palate. Gargle with flaxseed oil or
  another kind of nut or seed oil for a few minutes to rinse
  away any toxins in the gums and to protect against gum
  disease. Not all toxins will dissolve by gargling with just
  water so gargle with oil regularly.

* **Do thirty minutes of exercise:** try to incorporate at least
  thirty minutes of exercise per day. This may seem like a
  daunting task, but even something as simple as taking the
  stairs rather than the elevator contributes to your thirty
  minutes. Exercise comes in many different forms—a brisk
  walk, a bike ride, a game of tennis, a yoga class, a swim—so
  it shouldn't be difficult to find something that works for
  you and your lifestyle.

* **Keep hydrated:** by drinking water, vegetable tea or herbal
  tea throughout the day, you can keep your body properly
  hydrated. Aim to drink at least half a gallon a day, or more.
  Keep your vegetable tea on hand so you have something
  refreshing and nutritious to enjoy.

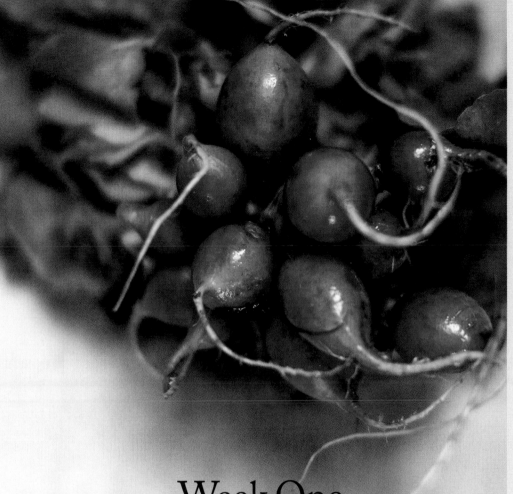

Week One

Week one's aim is to cleanse the system of toxins with a minimum of stress on the system. The menu is designed to bring the digestive system back into harmony, focusing on simple foods and smaller portions. The planner also includes daily exercises and beauty and environment tips for every other day.

WEEK ONE SHOPPING LIST

The shopping list below is to help you organize your first week of meals based on the menus we've listed in the day planner. The following list is for one person. If you are feeding more, increase proportionally.

Fresh Basics
These are fresh foods you will use through the week so buy as needed

Fresh herbs: parsley, rosemary, sage, thyme, basil, mint, lovage, cilantro, dill, nettle, yarrow, lemon balm, lemon verbena, chamomile and bay leaves

*

Vegetables, fruits and roots: ginger root, potatoes, fennel, juniper berries, turnips, celery, broccoli, green onions, zucchini, fresh horseradish, lemon, carrots, and parsnips

*

Milk products: milk (or soy milk or almond milk), curd, plain yogurt, goat's or sheep's cheese and butter

*

Other: eggs, spelt bread and crispbread

Days One and Two

1 chicken breast (3 oz)

*

4 baby potatoes

*

Green beans

*

Salad leaves

*

Parmesan (grated)

*

1 eggplant

*

Pitted black olives

Days Three and Four

1 tuna fillet (3 oz)

*

1 beef fillet (3 oz)

*

1 avocado

*

1 lime

*

1 sweet potato

*

1 apple

*

1 baking potato

*

Currants

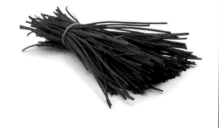

Days Five, Six and Seven

1 salmon fillet (3 oz)

*

1 avocado

*

1 apple

*

1 beet

*

1 eggplant

*

1 can of lima beans

*

Pitted black olives

*

Spinach

*

1 tomato

*

Dill

*

Currants

*

Chives

DAY ONE
Sunday

Take it slowly. One step at a time. You do not need to change the world before six o'clock. Give yourself a chance to welcome new ideas and get into a new mood, a new rhythm. Take your time. Calm is good. Speed is stressful. Put the brakes on…

WAKE UP
Hot water with lemon or
Rosemary Tea

BREAKFAST
Mediterranean Vegetable Spread
on spelt toast or crispbread

LUNCH
Grilled Chicken with Baby
Potatoes, Broccoli and Carrots

DINNER
Alkaline Minestrone

BEDTIME
Lemon Balm Tea

Cardio Exercise

Regular cardio exercise is an important part of the Alkaline Cure. Today, go for a brisk walk. Your pace should be fast enough that you feel your heart beating and your respiratory rate elevating. Try to walk at this pace for half an hour.

Beauty – Avocado Hair Mask

In a bowl, peel and mash a ripe avocado. Mix in a tablespoon of honey. Apply the mix to your hair and cover your head with a showercap. Leave the hair mask on for twenty minutes and then rinse out in the shower. This mask will leave your hair looking and feeling lustrous.

In the Kitchen

Soak your figs in hot herbal tea for breakfast

Liquidize your Vegetable Minestrone so it is a puree for tomorrow

Make your Almond Pesto

Prepare your Mayr Vegetable Tea

"Awareness is the conscious focusing on the moment. Perception and acceptance make us view the world as if it's in slow motion. Our environment and our own reactions become clearer."

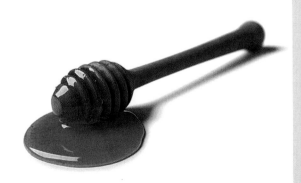

DAY TWO
Monday

Chewing is crucial to getting the most out of your food. It is a fundamental part of the Alkaline Cure. The quality of your chewing should make up for the smaller quantity of food. The better you chew, the better you will ingest and get all the nutrients from your food. Try to chew each mouthful thirty times.

WAKE UP
Hot water with lemon or
Ginger Tea

BREAKFAST
Fresh Yogurt with Flaxseed
Figs Poached in Herbal Tea

LUNCH
Salad of Green Beans, Potatoes
and Mixed Leaves in Olive Oil

DINNER
Smooth Alkaline Minestrone
Almond Pesto

BEDTIME
Lemon Balm Tea

Stretching – Stomach Exercise

This stretch is good for your core stomach muscles because it changes the pivotal point in the stomach. It also puts a different kind of pressure on the gut and works like an internal massage.

Lying down on your back, bring your knees up against your chest, then rotate your body—knees to the left, head to the right. Alternate.

Environment

Listen to calming, enjoyable music—perhaps something choral or classical. Maybe find a new theme to listen to in the evenings that you enjoy. Discover new composers and genres to go with your diet.

In the Kitchen

Make your Celery Soup
Soak your figs in hot herbal tea for breakfast

"Even the most alkaline recipes will turn acid in your stomach if you do not chew. Food should be savored and enjoyed slowly."

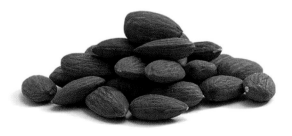

DAY THREE
Tuesday

The old saying was you should breakfast like a king, lunch like a prince and dine like a pauper. You can be a little lavish in the morning because your body has all day to digest, but be careful not to eat too much or you will make yourself feel hungrier later. The more you give your stomach, the more it wants. Give it less.

WAKE UP
Hot water with lemon or
Thyme Tea

BREAKFAST
Power Muesli
Figs Poached in Herbal Tea

LUNCH
Seared Tuna, Avocado, Ginger,
Cilantro and Lime

DINNER
Celery Soup

BEDTIME
Yarrow Tea

Relaxation – Breathing Exercise

This is a gentle breathing exercise that will calm both your mind and your spirit.

Sit in a comfortable, upright position and bring one hand close to your mouth, with the thumb and index fingers together, as if holding the end of a feather. Purse your lips and inhale slowly through your mouth. Then blow out gently, making a soft "hoo" sound, as if blowing an imaginary feather. Your fingertips should feel a cool breeze.

Repeat until you feel very calm and cool.

Beauty – Alkaline Bath

Top up your normal bath with one cup baking soda. With a pH indicator, check the water for a pH of 8.5. Soak for thirty to sixty minutes. As your skin wrinkles it will become soft and allow the acids to get out. This treatment is often used to treat arthritis and rheumatic diseases.

In the Kitchen

Assemble your Omega Mix
Prepare your Mayr
   Vegetable Tea

"If you feel like sitting down on the sofa after eating, that is a bad sign, a sign that you are eating the wrong things. After a meal, you should feel light, alert, full of energy."

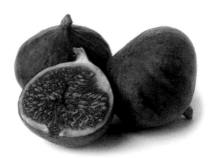

DAY FOUR
Wednesday

Change is good, for both the mind and the body. Exercise to move parts of the body you have forgotten about, especially the core. This is the new you.

WAKE UP
Hot water with lemon or
Sage Tea

BREAKFAST
Fresh Yogurt with Honey and
Omega Mix

LUNCH
Fillet of Beef with
Braised Celery and
Mashed Sweet Potato

DINNER
Baked Potato with Butter and Chives

BEDTIME
Yarrow Tea

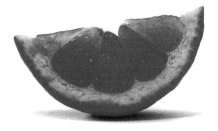

Strengthening – Core Exercise

This exercise will strengthen your core and improve your breathing by opening your chest.

Sit on the floor with your knees bent to the left side of your body and tuck your feet close to your right hip. Place your right foot into the arch of your left foot. Lengthen your spine, sit up tall and turn your torso to the left. Reach across your body with your right arm and place it on your left knee. Stretch your left arm behind you and place it on the floor. Untwist into the center position.

Repeat three times before changing directions.

Environment

Buy some colorful flowers and place them around your home where you can appreciate them: in the bathroom, your bedroom and the kitchen.

In the Kitchen

Make your Alkaline
   Minestrone
Prepare your Mediterranean
   Vegetable Spread
Soak your figs in hot herbal
   tea for breakfast

"If you move, you breathe off the acids building up in your body. The lungs ventilate; the acids offload. Motion is key. Any kind of motion is positive."

DAY FIVE
Thursday

Eating is about quality not quantity. The right foods at the right time. Take your time when eating: put your knife and fork down between mouthfuls, appreciate what you are doing. Allow yourself a good amount of time to eat, too—at least thirty minutes eating time, not including preparation.

WAKE UP
Hot water with lemon or
Peppermint Tea

BREAKFAST
Figs Poached in Herbal Tea
Mediterranean Vegetable Spread
on spelt toast or crispbread

LUNCH
Quinoa Salad with Avocado, Tomato,
Parsley and Pine Nuts
Olive Oil Dressing

DINNER
Alkaline Minestrone

BEDTIME
Chamomile Tea

Cardio Exercise

If you have a pool or a swimming complex nearby, go for a half-hour swim. Swimming is a low-impact cardio activity that works many muscle groups at once, stretching and strengthening your muscles. In the water, try different strokes and kicks. Swimming is not only good for your heart and muscles, it can also relieve sore joints.

Beauty – Sea Salt Scrub

Mix Dead Sea salt and almond oil together and gently exfoliate your body. Rinse with warm water and pat dry. Salt scrubs remove dead skin cells and bacteria, improve circulation and encourage cell regeneration.

In the Kitchen

Prepare your Sheep's Cheese and Horseradish Spread
Make your Herb Soup
Prepare your Mayr Vegetable Tea

"Eat enough. Sufficiently. You can train your body to live on less. It does not need more. That is life prolonging in itself."

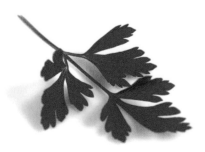

DAY SIX
Friday

Herbs come from the earth and so they bring with them their own minerality. Each herb has its own season and time of the year and makes its own contribution to your nutrition. Use them generously; they are valuable.

WAKE UP
Hot water with lemon or
Nettle Tea

BREAKFAST
Herb Omelet

LUNCH
Poached Salmon,
Carrot and Spinach Mash
and Hemp Sauce

DINNER
Herb Soup
Sheep's Cheese and Horseradish Spread
on spelt toast or crispbread

BEDTIME
Chamomile Tea

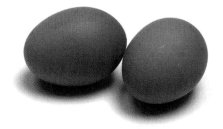

Stretching – Yoga Exercise

This yoga pose, called the Tree Pose, will help improve your balance, memory and concentration by engaging both your body and mind.

Stand in an upright position—feet firmly planted to the floor, knees locked, back straight and tall. Balance on one leg. Draw the opposite foot to the thigh or calf of the standing leg, never against the knee. Concentrate and raise your hands above your head. Remember to breathe; it will only interfere with your balance if you don't. Keep your hips even by lowering the position of your foot on your inner thigh.

Hold for five deep breaths then slowly come out of the posture. Alternate sides.

Environment

Switch off the television and your computer, and put your cell phone aside. Try to enjoy a relaxing evening without the buzz of the outside world.

In the Kitchen

Make your Spinach and Nutmeg Soup

"Bitterness is good. It is a sign of a natural, pure product—roots are bitter, and bitter plants like artichoke are helpful for the liver. So are radicchio and chicory. Herbs tend to be bitter. Dandelion is good, too, as are nettles in spring. Our liking for sweet things stems from our mother's milk, which was sweet. But as we get older, we need other things."

DAY SEVEN
Saturday

By now you should be feeling the benefits of changing your diet and enjoying lots of new foods and flavors—your body should also be feeling healthier and fitter. You have worked hard all week and have earned a relaxing day.

WAKE UP
Hot water with lemon or
Lemon Verbena Tea

BREAKFAST
Power Muesli

LUNCH
Roasted Beet, Lima Beans
and Chives with Walnut Oil

DINNER
Spinach and Nutmeg Soup

BEDTIME
Fennel Tea

Exercise
It's your seventh day and you've done well. This evening, take a relaxing stroll after dinner.

Treat
Take a steam at a sauna.

Beauty — Alkaline Footbath
Fill a small tub with warm water mixed with baking soda. Baking soda has many benefits, including skin smoothing and acting as an antifungal.

In the Kitchen
Make your Leek and Potato Soup
Prepare your Mayr Vegetable Tea
Soak your millet and buckwheat flakes

"You are your best doctor. I can only guide you. You know yourself better than I do. You know your body. You just have to be aware of bad influences. The more you can program yourself and your responses with alkaline messages, the easier it will become to identify and listen to what your body is saying. Listen to your body. Have a talk with it."

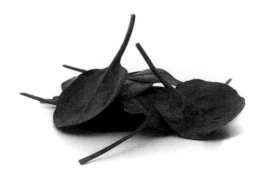

BUILDING ON YOUR CURE

After a week of gentle cleansing, your body should be responding and you may notice that what you are eating tastes better. In the past seven days, depending on your previous lifestyle, you may have experienced severe headaches, anxiety, mood changes and cravings. At the health center we usually say that it takes at least ten days for all of the benefits to start to kick in, but you should already begin to notice some positive changes happening after this first week. Generally, you should be feeling more energized, your skin should be looking clearer, and you should be feeling more regular and less constipated and bloated.

Balancing Week

For your second week we want to introduce some more ideas that will make cooking and eating more enjoyable and give you a head start to the alkaline way of life. While last week we were concerned with nursing your system back to health, this week we are looking to stimulate your body and mind and create a new kind of balance.

Little things matter. A scattering of sesame or sunflower seeds can spice up a breakfast; a drizzle of pumpkin oil or flaxseed oil can bring new elements to plain curd or yogurt. This week, make good use of your alkaline pantry and, with it, build up new levels of flavor and nutrition at every meal.

As you continue on with the plan, remember to keep yourself hydrated—half a gallon or more of water a day will help to wash out the toxins in your system and keep your body working properly.

Week Two

*For all of the cleansing foods we ate last week, this week we
can open up and explore some new and different foods. The recipes
are still easy to follow but use a wider spectrum of ingredients for
fuller, more creative meals. The more different alkaline foods
we eat, the more our bodies can take advantage
of the nutritional benefits they offer.*

WEEK TWO SHOPPING LIST

The shopping list below is to help you organize your second week of meals based on the menus we've listed in the day planner. The following list is for one person. If you are feeding more, increase proportionally.

Fresh Basics

These are fresh foods you will use throughout the week so buy as needed

Fresh herbs: parsley, rosemary, sage, thyme, basil, mint, lovage, cilantro, dill, nettle, yarrow, lemon balm, lemon verbena, chamomile and bay

*

Vegetables, fruits and roots: ginger root, potatoes, fennel, juniper berries, turnips, celery, broccoli, green onions, zucchini, fresh horseradish, lemon, carrots, and parsnips

*

Milk products: milk (or soy milk or almond milk), curd, plain yogurt, goat's or sheep's cheese and butter

*

Other: eggs, spelt bread and crispbread

Days Eight and Nine

Smoked mackerel (3 oz)

*

1 grapefruit

*

1 artichoke

*

2 shiitake mushrooms

*

10 snowpeas

*

5 leeks

*

1 bok choy

*

Lemongrass

*

Green beans

*

Coconut milk

*

Rice noodles or tofu

*

Cream or Crème fraîche

*

Chives

*

Mustard

Days Ten, Eleven and Twelve

Ground beef
(3 oz; buy on Day 11)
*
1 orange
*
1 grapefruit
*
Strawberries
*
1 avocado
*
1 red pepper
*
1 eggplant
*
1 sweet potato
*
1 garlic bulb
*
Pitted black olives
*
1 kohlrabi
*
1 celeriac
*
1 cucumber
*
Cream
*
3 chestnuts

Days Thirteen and Fourteen

1 lamb chop (3 oz)
*
1 lime
*
2 avocados
*
2 fresh figs
*
1 small melon of choice
*
Berries of choice
*
1 cucumber
*
1 beet

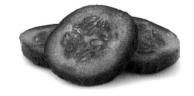

DAY EIGHT
Sunday

Today is a spice day. Historically, spices were used as medicine to spruce up the system. Many spices still form the basis of our modern medicine, and they bring benefits to your diet that may be neglected in your daily meals. In their natural form, they have a valuable role to play.

WAKE UP
Hot water with lemon or
Rosemary Tea

BREAKFAST
Millet and Buckwheat Porridge
with Cinnamon and Ginger

LUNCH
Asian-Style Stir-Fry

DINNER
Leek and Potato Soup

BEDTIME
Fennel Tea

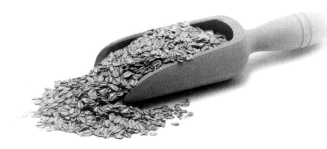

Relaxation – Breathing Exercise

Create your own breathing sequence using all three of these upper body breathing exercises: for abdomen, for chest and for shoulders. Try to do it outside or in front of an open window.

Sitting down with your back straight, put your fingers on your stomach. Breathe in hard with your belly so you can feel the effect on your diaphragm—your fingers should move apart. Repeat ten times, long and slow.

Sitting down with your back straight, bring your fingers up to your chest. Breathe in deeply, feel the strength of your lungs. Exhale slowly. Repeat ten times.

Place your hands on your collarbones and breathe in, concentrating on the whole of the upper body. Breathe out and relax. Repeat twenty times.

Environment	In the Kitchen
Turn off the alarm clock and let your body decide how much sleep you really need. Try to wake up naturally at dawn.	Prepare your Curd and Paprika Spread

"The only supplement I might recommend that you cannot always find in your diet is zinc. The importance of zinc is that it forces the body to produce bicarbonate naturally. However, it is mostly found in oysters and red meats. You can be low on zinc without noticing, although it is often seen in poor hair and brittle nails."

DAY NINE
Monday

The oils that you have been using throughout the week provide essential omegas in your diet. They are the switches that turn what we eat into nutrition. Blend and vary the oils you use. Flaxseed oil is the most valuable because it is high in omega-3 and makes a great base oil for mixes. But if you don't like the flavor of flaxseed oil, then other nut oils, olive oils and organic seed oils can be used as they are also immensely important.

WAKE UP
Hot water with lemon or
Ginger Tea

BREAKFAST
Grapefruit
Curd and Paprika Spread
on spelt toast or crispbread

LUNCH
Artichoke Hearts with Flaxseed
and Herb Vinaigrette

DINNER
Smoked Mackerel and
Vegetables with Parsley Oil

BEDTIME
Lemon Balm Tea

Strengthening – Core Exercise

This exercise will help improve your coordination, which plays a major role in core strengthening.

Kneel on your hands and knees, holding weights in both hands. Form a straight line from your shoulders to your hands and from your hips to your knees. Stretch one leg out straight behind your torso on the floor while stretching your opposite arm on the floor in front of you. Lift your extended arm and leg up to shoulder and hip level. Keep your palm down. Lower your arm and leg to the floor.

Lift and lower five times and then alternate sides.

Beauty – Warm Liver Compress

Apply a warm compress on your liver before you go to bed. Wrap a dampened tea towel around a hot water bottle filled with warm water. Lie back and place it underneath your ribs and to the right. Leave for fifteen minutes or even all night.

In the Kitchen

Make up your Carrot and
  Ginger Soup
Prepare your Mediterranean
  Vegetable Spread
Prepare your Mayr
  Vegetable Tea

*"Sweating is good. Train your body to sweat.
You are getting rid of the acids."*

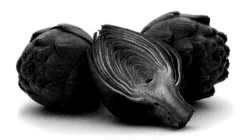

DAY TEN
Tuesday

Most of us have developed a habit of eating too much. Cut your portion sizes down. At restaurants, do not be tempted to eat everything on your plate. At home, use small plates rather than big ones. Mix up your diet with different things to keep meal times interesting. Eat slower so that you take the same amount of time for dinner but eat less. Put your cutlery down between mouthfuls.

WAKE UP
Hot water with lemon or
Thyme Tea

BREAKFAST
Fresh Yogurt with Honey and
Omega Mix

LUNCH
Baked Pepper Stuffed with Bulgur Wheat
and Nuts

DINNER
Carrot and Ginger Soup
Mediterranean Vegetable Spread
on spelt toast or crispbread

BEDTIME
Lemon Balm Tea

Cardio Exercise

Today, go for a jog or, if you have the equipment, use an elliptical for at least half an hour. Try to fluctuate your pace while jogging: every five minutes, increase your pace by thirty percent for a minute.

Environment

Buy some houseplants. They will improve the oxygen circulation in your rooms and lend a calming presence to your décor.

In the Kitchen

Soak your apricots in hot herbal tea for breakfast

Prepare your Herb Spread

"If you cannot sleep, treat it as an advantage. You have more time in the day. Relax and enjoy the sweet and tranquil rhythm of your thoughts. Watch them go by without interfering. Go with the flow. You do not need to sleep to be relaxed and rested."

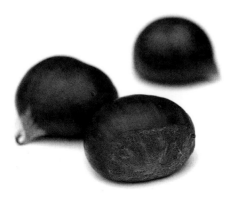

DAY ELEVEN
Wednesday

Keep up your routines—exercising, preparing meals, dry skin brushing, bathing, sleeping. Routine is an immensely strong thing. The body prepares itself better if things are regular. Hormones have a twenty-four-hour cycle and are easily disturbed. In order to reset their balance, you need to have a regular routine.

WAKE UP
Hot water with lemon or
Sage Tea

BREAKFAST
Goat's cheese on spelt toast or crispbread
Apricots Poached in Herbal Tea

LUNCH
Spicy Meatballs with Tzatziki
Strawberries

DINNER
Warm Salad of Kohlrabi,
Broccoli and Celeriac in Herb Oil
Herb Spread on spelt toast or crispbread

BEDTIME
Yarrow Tea

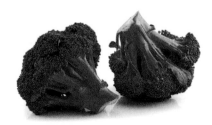

Relaxation – Breathing Exercise

Sit in a comfortable upright position. Close your eyes and breathe naturally. Rest your right hand on your right knee, keeping your hand relaxed and open.

Raise your left hand and place your thumb gently against your left nostril. Breathe in slowly, taking a full breath through your right nostril. Gently close your right nostril with the ring finger of your left hand. Hold for a second, then slowly release the ring finger and breathe out through your right nostril until your lungs are empty.

Repeat five times and then switch sides, inhaling and exhaling through your left nostril. Repeat five times.

Beauty – Alkaline Face Mask

You can make an easy alkaline face mask with curd or quark and honey. Honey is an antimicrobial and an antioxidant while curd soothes. Simply combine the two, apply and leave for ten minutes before rinsing.

In the Kitchen

Make your Fennel and
    Dill Soup
Prepare your Herb Spread
    (if needed)
Prepare your Mayr
    Vegetable Tea

"Breathing helps to make us aware of our bodies. It helps us to focus on the core, the abdomen, the torso and not always think of our bodies as arms and legs. Even in the office, take five minutes, open a window, put your hands on your knees, and breathe in at different tempos—fast like laughing, slow and deep to create rhythm. Follow your heartbeat, remember who you are."

DAY TWELVE
Thursday

As you near the end of your fourteen-day plan, your body should be enjoying its natural rhythms and processes. You should be starting to feel less stressed, more energized and more positive. You will find that eating alkaline is starting to become second nature, rather than a regime you have to adhere to. You will start to associate healthy food with feeling good and stop craving the unhealthy foods you may have craved before.

WAKE UP
Hot water with lemon or
Peppermint Tea

BREAKFAST
Grapefruit
Millet and Buckwheat Porridge
with Cinnamon and Ginger

LUNCH
Quinoa Risotto

DINNER
Fennel and Dill Soup
Herb Spread on spelt toast or crispbread

BEDTIME
Yarrow Tea

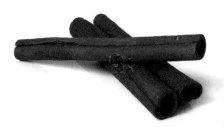

Strengthening – Core Exercise

This exercise, called spine curls, requires you to peel your spine off of the floor vertebra by vertebra. Doing these slowly will help further strengthen your core.

Lie flat on your back with your knees bent and your feet on the floor hip-width apart. Breathe in. As you breathe out, tilt your pelvis so that your lower back sinks into the mat and your pubic bone lifts toward the ceiling. Breathe in. Breathe out as you lower yourself back down.

Repeat, lifting a little more of your spine off the floor each time until you have lifted your whole abdomen up to your shoulder blades. Hold the position and breathe in. As you breathe out, gently reverse the movement.

Environment

You have cleaned your system, now clean out your home. Get rid of things you don't need and establish an orderly living environment.

In the Kitchen

Prepare your Sheep's Cheese and Horseradish Spread

"Turn off all the electronics in your bedroom. The best light for us is still candlelight. Our ancestors gathered around an open fire to meet and to talk and that is still the most positive kind of light we are attuned to."

DAY THIRTEEN
Friday

Listen to your body's rhythms and learn to adapt to a better lifestyle. Your body will naturally tell you what it needs, but you have to recognize the good signals and not slip back into bad habits. For instance, if your body feels tired and you're not at work or doing something important, lie down and have a nap. Be a friend to yourself and your body.

WAKE UP
Hot water with lemon or
Nettle Tea

BREAKFAST
Melon
Sheep's Cheese and Horseradish Spread
on spelt toast or crispbread

LUNCH
Gratin of Potatoes, Onion and Nutmeg

DINNER
Roasted Beet with Walnut Oil and Caraway Seeds
Braised Fennel with Zucchini

BEDTIME
Chamomile Tea

Cardio Exercise

Today, go for a bike ride either on a bike outside or on a stationary bike. Aim to go for half an hour and try to challenge yourself with different inclines and gears. Cycling will tone and strengthen your legs, thighs and glutes. It is a lower impact activity than running and it can also relieve back pain and muscle strain in your feet and knees.

Beauty – Milk and Honey Bath

Add half a gallon of milk and one cup of honey to a warm bath. Soak for at least fifteen minutes. Afterward, your skin will radiate and feel like silk.

In the Kitchen

Prepare your Mayr
  Vegetable Tea
Make your
  Alkaline Minestrone
Prepare your Avocado Spread

"Potassium is essential in pushing out the acids through the body. As soon as you are alkaline, the vegetables you eat facilitate the benefits to the body."

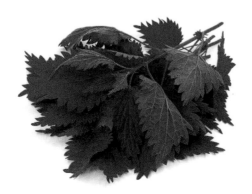

DAY FOURTEEN
Saturday

Well done! You should be feeling energized and revitalized—a new you. Enjoy your new vitality and reflect on all the changes you have made in the past two weeks. Don't beat yourself up if there are still things you wish to change. Remember, you are you, and now you're off to a wonderful new start. Remember to keep going and you will surprise yourself with how good you can feel.

WAKE UP
Hot water with lemon or
Lemon Verbena Tea

BREAKFAST
Fresh berries and melon
Avocado Spread on spelt toast or crispbread

LUNCH
Grilled Lamb Chop with
Fennel, Cucumber, Grapefruit and Fig Salad

DINNER
Alkaline Minestrone

BEDTIME
Chamomile Tea

Exercise

As a reward for your hard work these past two weeks, take a gentle stroll this evening and enjoy your alkaline body.

Treat

Get a reflexology massage. The massage focuses on reflex areas on your feet that are connected to parts of your body in order to relax these areas and open the energy flow. It promotes circulation and general healing.

"Modern life is acid. Accept it. See it for what it is and you can have your life back. You don't have to give up everything. You will just find some better alternatives, that is all. Enjoy it."

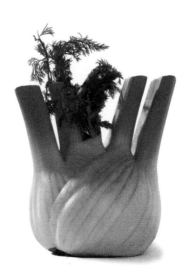

AFTER THE CURE

There are many things to take away after finishing the Alkaline Cure. Perhaps, after cleansing, you have lost some weight or you find yourself more agile physically and mentally. You may feel more supple, have fewer aches and pains. As you can see, a few small changes can have a dramatic effect and are more achievable than trying to change everything in an afternoon or even a month. Remember, a good regime is not just for fourteen days. The Alkaline Cure is a way of life, not a one-off detox. Keep going and you may surprise yourself with how good you can feel.

Hopefully you will have picked up enough tips to keep your system in balance, and hopefully you enjoyed it. Don't forget to slow down, chew well and really enjoy what you are eating. Listen to your body and eat only what will make your body feel good and healthy. Try to keep up your exercise at least every other day—it doesn't matter so much what you do for exercise but rather that you exercise in the first place. And, in the whirlwind of everyday life, try to give yourself a good, manageable routine. With positive routines, your body will generate more power and energy.

A Regular Cure

Regularly repeating the Alkaline Cure will help you to establish a new self-understanding and build up your discipline. However, because you and your body have changed, your experiences each time around will feel slightly different.

Curing should become a part of your annual routine. It should be like—as it is for many people who come to the health center each year—a summer holiday. Annually book yourself back into the Alkaline Cure, but instead give yourself three weeks of cleansing. Hopefully by then many of the principles in this book will be an integral part of your everyday life, and you will be feeling the life-changing benefits.

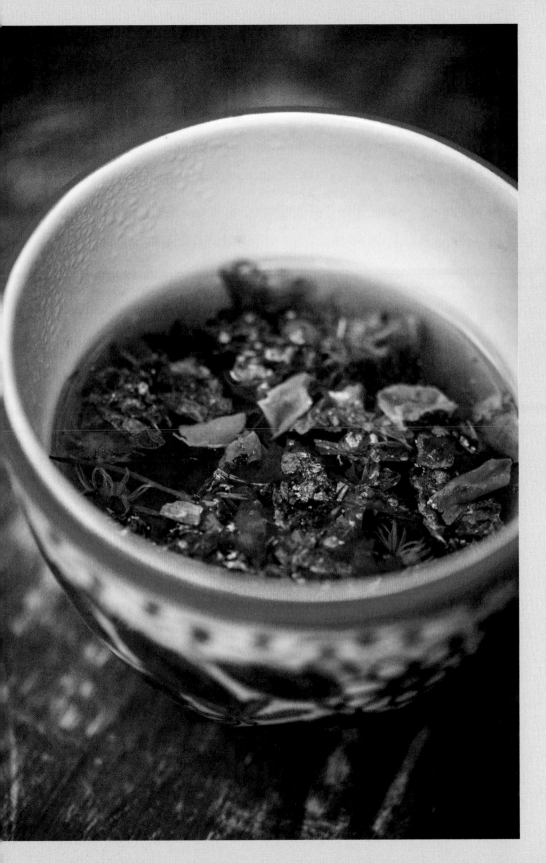

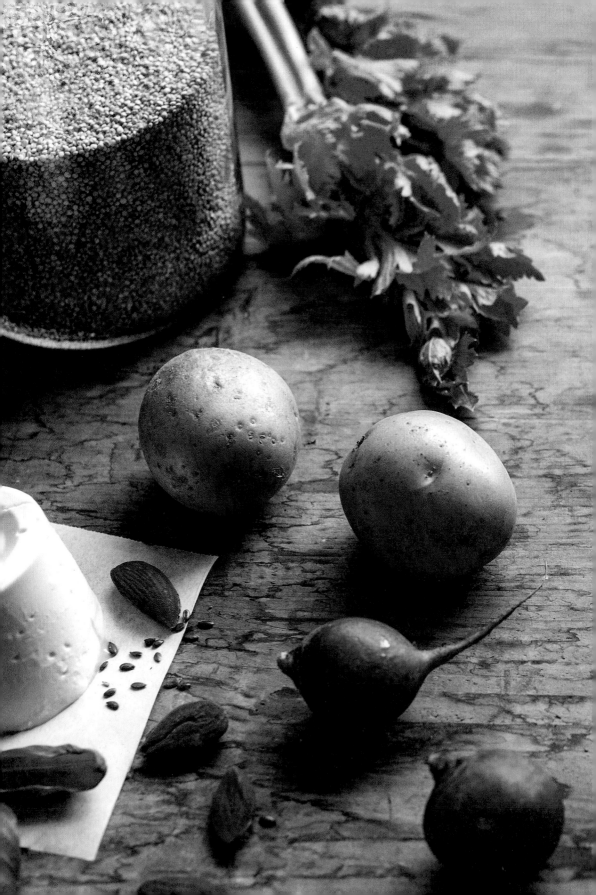

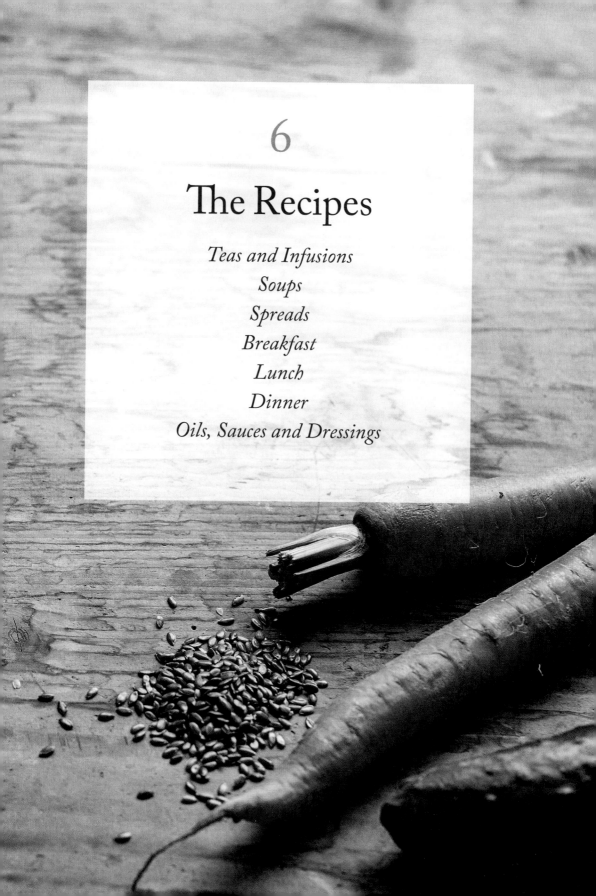

6

The Recipes

Teas and Infusions
Soups
Spreads
Breakfast
Lunch
Dinner
Oils, Sauces and Dressings

TEAS AND INFUSIONS

Teas and infusions are an excellent way of ensuring your body gets enough liquid through the day. They also offer many other health benefits. Though we recommend the following teas, there are many other great alkaline teas that you can substitute, such as rosehip, lavender, redbush and yerba mate. When making your own herbal tea infusions with fresh herbs or roots, simply add one cup of boiling water to one tablespoon of fresh herbs (or one teaspoon of dried herbs or grated root). Infuse the herbs for up to three minutes and strain.

MAYR VEGETABLE TEA

You can mix up the alkaline vegetables and spices according to the season. Rhubarb is a good addition, too, if you cannot find lovage. Drink this tea throughout the day to stay hydrated.

4 cups water	1 tablespoon lovage, chopped
1 carrot, chopped	
1 celery stalk, chopped	1 tablespoon parsley, chopped
1 potato, chopped	
Half a fennel bulb, chopped	1 tablespoon fennel seeds
1 broccoli stalk, chopped	1 teaspoon coriander seeds
Parsley stalks	1 teaspoon cumin seeds
1 teaspoon juniper berries	4 bay leaves

Put a large saucepan of cold water on to boil. Simmer the vegetables for ten minutes and then add your spices. Cover and simmer for 30 minutes. Turn off the heat. Leave to cool and infuse for another ten minutes.

Strain and keep the tea for use through the day—hot or cold.

MORNING TEAS

Your body is tuned to digest after a night's sleep. To get it started, a cup of hot water with (or without) a squeeze of lemon or lime first thing is the equivalent of rubbing the sleep out of your eyes. Drink this half an hour before breakfast. You can also enjoy the following morning teas to get you up and ready for the coming day.

Rosemary
Rosemary is an energizing herb, known to promote blood circulation. It also stimulates digestion and improves cognitive function.

Ginger
Ginger tea is known for its ability to ease digestion and reduce nausea, but it has a number of other benefits as well. Packed with antioxidants, ginger also reduces inflammation, fights respiratory problems and relieves stress. Ginger increases blood circulation as well, which accounts for the warming sensation you experience when you drink it.

Thyme
Thyme is a remarkable herb. Not only can it clear chest congestion, relieve gas and bloating, and act as a diuretic, it is also full of antioxidants and essential minerals, such as iron, vitamin K, manganese and calcium.

Sage
Sage is loaded with antioxidants. Antioxidants defend your body against harmful free radicals, which attack your cells and can lead to heart disease, cancer and premature aging. Sage also relieves inflammation and treats gastrointestinal problems.

Peppermint
Peppermint tea is known to ease digestion and settle upset stomachs and nausea. It also contains calcium, vitamin B and potassium, which boost your immune system. Peppermint tea also has a calming effect and therefore works as a great evening tea as well.

Nettle

Nettle has antiseptic and antimicrobial properties. It also contains many essential vitamins and minerals—such as iron, potassium and magnesium—as well as phytochemicals, which attack many of the free radicals that come from our environments. However, be careful not to consume too much nettle tea, as it can have an effect on blood sugar, blood pressure, anxiety, insomnia and blood clotting—especially if you are taking medication for any of these conditions.

Lemon Verbena

Lemon verbena has a calming effect on the nervous system and can even battle stress and symptoms of depression. The herb also aids digestion and helps relieve intestinal problems, such as nausea and diarrhea.

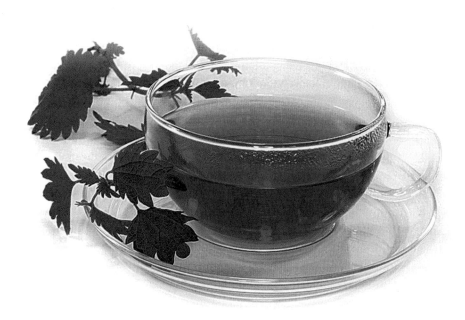

EVENING TEAS

After you've finished dinner and your daily tasks, relax and unwind with an evening tea. The following teas are know for their ability to ease digestion and calm your body, priming you for a good night's rest.

Lemon Balm

Lemon balm is a great evening tea because of its ability to calm. It treats everything from nervous agitation and digestive upsets to heart palpitations and viral infections. Lemon balm is also sleep-inducing, so try a cup before you turn in for the night.

Yarrow

Historically, yarrow was used for treating and healing wounds, but it has a number of other functions. Yarrow helps the body to sweat by relaxing the skin's pores and increasing blood circulation. It is also used to treat digestive issues—it stimulates the bowels and relieves gas and cramps.

Chamomile

Chamomile is best known as a sleep aid and, therefore, works well as a relaxing evening tea. It also soothes stomach and digestive issues while regulating digestion. Chamomile is antibacterial and can be used to treat wounds and fight colds.

Fennel

You can make this tea with either the fennel's seeds, feathery leaves, roots or a combination of all three. It needs to be drunk right away to catch all the more volatile compounds before they evaporate. Fennel tea has long been known to help with digestive issues, relieving cramps and flatulence. It also acts as a diuretic, relieves pains and has antimicrobial properties.

SOUPS

Soup does not have to be just soup and you can make it more interesting by adding fresh herbs or flaxseed, nut or olive oils before serving. Liquidize your soup to make it creamier and easier to digest. Soups are also useful for bringing important vegetables into your diet in different ways. They can be made the night before and either taken to work or reheated when you get home. And since soups need a bit of time to improve, it is a good idea to make them ahead anyways.

❶ ALKALINE MINESTRONE

This is our basic soup recipe, and the yield will last for a few days. It can be slipped into the diet for lunch or dinner. It is hearty, nutritious, healthy and delicious. By all means, vary the vegetables with the season and top up the soup with water you have used to cook other vegetables. This soup will last two or three days, and, if you eat nothing else, it is a big step forward to an alkaline way of life.

4 cups water or organic vegetable stock	1 turnip, chopped
	1 celery stalk, chopped
1 medium potato, peeled and chopped	⅓ cup diced green onions
	⅔ cup fresh cream
1 carrot, chopped	Rock or sea salt
1 parsnip, chopped	

In a large saucepan, bring four cups of water or stock to a simmer. Add the chopped potato. Add the other vegetables to the pot. Boil for about 15 minutes or until the vegetables are soft.

Turn off the heat and pour carefully into a food processor or use an electric handheld blender. Add the cream and the rock or sea salt to taste. Blend into a puree and garnish.

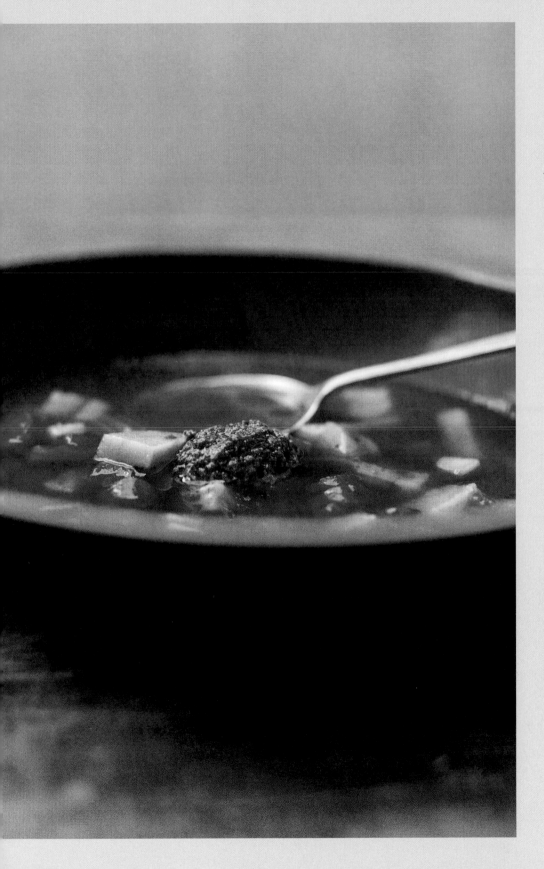

❶ CELERY SOUP

1 head of celery, chopped	1 bunch parsley,
1 potato, peeled and	roughly chopped
chopped	1 tablespoon curd
4 cups water	Rock or sea salt

Chop the celery and potato into small chunks. Add the celery and potato to four cups of water and simmer for 20 minutes. Add in just the stalks from the parsley, keeping the fronds as a garnish.

When the vegetables are soft, remove the heat and liquidize the soup with a food processor or hand blender until smooth. Season to taste with rock or sea salt. Dice the parsley heads and scatter on the soup along with a tablespoon of fresh curd.

❶ HERB SOUP

Herb soups are a great way to maximize the herbs you have in your garden or fridge, especially parsley, lovage and sorrel. The soup can also be filled out with a little spinach. In order to get a good, green color, add the leaves in the food processor without cooking. However, the stalks of parsley and cilantro should go in at the start to flavor the broth. Use a good mix of herbs for this soup.

2 medium potatoes,	Herbs: parsley, basil,
peeled and chopped	chervil, lovage, cilantro,
4 cups water or organic	thyme, rosemary
vegetable stock	Ground nutmeg
	Rock or sea salt

Boil the potatoes in water or vegetable stock until tender. Blend in a food processor or with an electric handheld blender. Add fresh herbs and blend again until the soup has a bright green color. Add nutmeg and season with rock or sea salt.

Ⓥ SPINACH AND NUTMEG SOUP

This is the fastest soup we know and it is also bursting with iron. You can give it new dimensions by adding herbs like parsley, cilantro or dill. You can probably also allow yourself a knob of butter or a touch of cream without upsetting the soup's alkalinity.

> 4 cups water or organic vegetable stock
> 2 cups fresh organic spinach
> Rock or sea salt
> Nutmeg

Bring the water or vegetable stock to a boil in a large saucepan. Add washed spinach. Boil for one minute at most. Blend the soup in a food processor until smooth. Season to taste with rock or sea salt and a grating of nutmeg.

Ⓥ LEEK AND POTATO SOUP

Leek and potato soup, sometimes called vichyssoise *when more cream is used, is both classic and also excellently alkaline. Traditionally, it is served cold in the summer and hot in the winter.*

> 2 tablespoons butter
> 1 medium onion, skinned and diced
> 4 potatoes, peeled and diced
> 4 leeks, finely chopped
> 4 cups water or organic vegetable stock
> 1 cup milk
> Rock or sea salt
> Pepper
> Fresh chives or parsley, chopped
> 4 tablespoons of cream or crème fraîche (optional)

Melt the butter in a large saucepan and add the onion to cook until translucent, then add the potato and the leeks and stir well. After five minutes, add the vegetable stock and the milk and cook for another 20 minutes. Season with salt and pepper. Liquidize if you wish. Garnish with chopped chives, parsley or a spoon of cream.

❶ CARROT AND GINGER SOUP

3 cups carrots, washed
and chopped
1 small potato, washed
and chopped

3 cups water or organic
vegetable stock
1 small ginger root
1 orange
Rock or sea salt
Parsley

Juice one-third of the carrots. Boil the remaining carrots and potatoes in vegetable stock or water until tender. Blend in a food processor until smooth. Grate in enough ginger to season. Add the carrot juice and season with rock or sea salt. Add a squeeze of orange and garnish with parsley.

❶ FENNEL AND DILL SOUP

This soup was originally the recipe F.X. Mayr used to train patients to chew properly along with his famous spelt bread. It is simple and easy to make and very distinct. This soup is to be eaten slowly. And be sure to be generous with the herbs.

4 cups water or organic vegetable stock
1 fennel bulb, cut into four segments
1 bunch dill
Rock or sea salt

Bring the water or vegetable stock to a boil in a medium pot. Dice three of the fennel segments and add to the water or stock. Juice the remaining segment and set aside.

When the fennel is cooked—just soft, about 12 minutes—add it to the food processor. Add in the fennel juice and the dill. Blend until smooth and season with rock or sea salt.

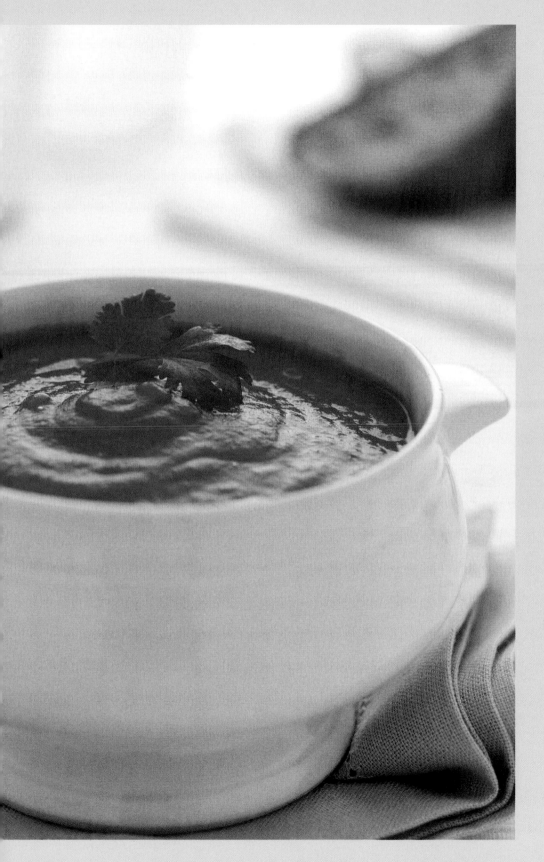

SPREADS

The following alkaline spreads are nutrient-dense alternatives to your traditional breakfast spreads, such as jam or peanut butter, which can be both high in sugar and salt and loaded with preservatives. They are versatile and easy to make, and the ingredients can be combined in countless ways. Enjoy the spreads over crispbread or spelt toast. Have one slice of crispbread or toast per meal and save the rest of your spread for the next day. You can substitute in quark, cottage cheese or probiotic yogurt if you don't have curd.

ⓥ MEDITERRANEAN VEGETABLE SPREAD

One-quarter of a small
    eggplant, chopped
Half a zucchini, chopped
¼ cup pitted black olives
¼ cup yogurt

⅔ cup fresh, soft sheep's
    or goat's cheese
2 tablespoons fresh basil
Rock or sea salt
Olive oil

Heat a few drops of olive oil in a nonstick frying pan. Sweat the eggplant for two or three minutes. Then add the zucchini and cook for another two minutes. Blend in a food processor with the olives, yogurt and cheese. Season with rock or sea salt. Finish with the basil. Add a little virgin olive oil if needed.

ⓥ SHEEP'S CHEESE AND HORSERADISH SPREAD

½ cup fresh soft
    sheep's or goat's cheese
1 small potato,
    cooked and pressed

1 teaspoon fresh grated
    horseradish
1 teaspoon fresh dill,
    finely chopped
Pinch of rock or sea salt

Blend all the ingredients in a food processor until very fine and season with rock or sea salt.

⊙ CURD AND PAPRIKA SPREAD

¼ cup fresh curd cheese
1 tablespoon paprika
1 tablespoon flaxseed oil

Sprinkle paprika and drizzle flaxseed oil over the curd. Mix
to combine.

⊙ HERB SPREAD

¼ cup curd or fresh goat's
or sheep's cheese
1 tablespoon flaxseed or
olive oil
1 tablespoon parsley,
finely chopped

1 tablespoon chives,
finely chopped
1 tablespoon cilantro,
finely chopped
Paprika

Using the back of a fork, mash the curd or cheese with the flaxseed
or olive oil. Mix the herbs into the mashed curd. Dust with paprika.
Leave for five minutes to macerate.

⊙ AVOCADO SPREAD

2 ripe avocados
1 cup sheep's cheese curd
Juice of half a lime
1 teaspoon basil,
finely shredded

1 tablespoon sesame seeds
Pinch of rock or sea salt
Olive or pumpkin oil

Peel the avocados by cutting through the skin at quarter intervals and
peeling back the skin. Mash or blend the avocado flesh. Mix well with
the curd and the juice of the lime. Add the shredded basil and the
sesame seeds. Season with rock or sea salt. Add a drizzle of virgin olive
or pumpkin oil. Serve immediately.

BREAKFAST

Breakfast can be one of the most important changes a person makes to their diet while on the Alkaline Cure. Breakfast should be a point where you bring in a wide range of different alkaline foods, particularly raw foods, because you have a whole day ahead to digest. Spreads are a great way of doing this and, therefore, should become a solid breakfast staple as well. The following recipes typically serve one.

ⓥ DRIED FRUIT POACHED IN HERBAL TEA

The alkaline triumvirate of dried apricots, figs and prunes can be given an extra boost by soaking them in herbal tea. They are a refreshing, nutritious hit to start the morning. You can drink the tea, too, which is delicious. Vary both the type of herbal tea and dried fruit, as you like.

1 cup dried apricots, prunes or figs
1 tablespoon herbal tea of your choice
Water

Boil the water. Place the apricots, prunes, and figs in a bowl. Pour over the boiled water. Add the herbs. Leave to cool and then store in the refrigerator.

ⓥ FRESH YOGURT WITH FLAXSEED

½ cup of fresh yogurt
1 tablespoon flaxseed
1 tablespoon flaxseed oil

Sprinkle flaxseed and drizzle flaxseed oil over the yogurt.
Mix to combine.

Fresh Yogurt with Honey and Omega Mix
Sprinkle a tablespoon of Omega Mix (opposite) over the fresh yogurt. Sweeten with a teaspoon of honey. Make this breakfast more alkaline with the juice of a lemon.

◉ POWER MUESLI

Muesli can be difficult to digest so it is a good idea to soak it the night before in milk, apple juice, a thin yogurt, soy milk or almond milk. In the morning, mix with fresh fruit, soaked dried fruits (such as raisins), seeds, and nuts— especially almonds, for an even broader range of vitamins. This recipe will be enough for two or three breakfasts.

2 tablespoons oats	½ tablespoon walnut oil
2 tablespoons millet flakes	½ tablespoon flax oil
2 tablespoons buckwheat flakes	One-quarter of an apple
	Half a carrot
1 cup almond milk, milk or apple juice	1 inch celery, diced
	1 tablespoon currants
1 tablespoon sheep's yogurt	1 tablespoon crushed almonds

Soak the oats, millet, and buckwheat in almond milk, milk, or apple juice. Add in the raisins and leave overnight. In the morning, grate in the apple and carrot. Dice the celery and add it in. Top with the yogurt, oils and almonds.

◉ OMEGA MIX

You can get the benefits of seeds by creating your own mix in a coffee grinder or food processor. This mix is perfect for sprinkling on porridge, muesli, or salads.

3 parts flaxseed
1 part pumpkin seeds
1 part sesame seeds
1 part sunflower seeds

Mix together and grind before use. You can store the mix in a jar and keep in either your pantry or your fridge.

ⓥ MILLET AND BUCKWHEAT PORRIDGE WITH CINNAMON AND GINGER

This recipe is a simpler variation on porridge that brings in some valuable spices.

⅓ cup millet flakes
⅓ cup buckwheat flakes
2 cups milk, soy milk
   or almond milk

1 teaspoon cinnamon
1 tablespoon grated ginger
1 tablespoon maple syrup

Soak the millet and buckwheat flakes in milk either overnight or for at least ten minutes. On the stove, bring the porridge to a bubble, stirring and allowing it to thicken. Powder over with cinnamon and grate the ginger on top. Add the maple syrup.

ⓥ HERB OMELET

Eggs can be an easy source of protein, once or twice a week. The yolk is, after all, alkaline. Here, they are the perfect medium for fresh herbs.

2 eggs
Half a bunch of parsley,
chopped finely

Half a bunch of chives,
   chopped finely
Rock or sea salt
Butter

Warm a nonstick frying pan and melt a knob of butter in it. Break the eggs into a cup and beat with a pinch of rock or sea salt. Pour the beaten eggs into the hot frying pan. As the omelet cooks, chop your herbs finely. Once the omelet begins to set, add the herbs, covering the omelet well. Fold over the omelet and leave to cook for a minute until set.

LUNCH

Lunch is the best time to explore a fuller range of alkaline ingredients. Your body still has a good amount of time to digest properly and, therefore you are safe to incorporate both raw and cooked foods. The following recipes are much more interesting than your typical brown-bag lunch, and far more alkaline, too. Each recipe typically serves one.

GRILLED CHICKEN WITH BABY POTATOES, BROCCOLI AND CARROTS

3 oz chicken breast
4 baby potatoes, chopped
2 broccoli florets and
   their stalks
2 tablespoons almonds
1 carrot, chopped

1 tablespoon butter
2 tablespoons cilantro,
   chopped
2 tablespoons mint, chopped
Rock or sea salt

Turn on the grill to warm up. Trim the broccoli so you have florets. In a tiered steamer, put the potatoes on to steam first, then add the carrots and broccoli stalks. Grill the chicken for five minutes. Turn over and grill for five more minutes. In a dry frying pan, toast the almonds quickly until they just begin to change color—you can smell this happening.

Add your broccoli florets after ten minutes to the potatoes and other vegetables. After another five minutes, drain the vegetables, adding the cooking water to your minestrone stock or your vegetable tea. Plate your grilled chicken.

Toss the vegetables in the butter until melted and arrange them around the meat. Sprinkle the almonds over the broccoli, the cilantro over the carrots and the mint over the potatoes. Season with salt.

❶ SALAD OF GREEN BEANS, POTATOES AND MIXED LEAVES IN OLIVE OIL

This is an easy, quick and nutritious lunch that is bulked up by the vegetables from your minestrone. You can vary the other vegetables as you like. Remember to top your soups up with the cooking water from your vegetables.

⅔ cup green beans, trimmed

1 small potato, washed and chopped

½ cup mixed vegetables from your minestrone

3 cups mixed salad leaves

1½ tablespoons sunflower or sesame seeds

Pumpkin Oil Dressing (page 168)

Place the potatoes in a tiered steamer. Steam for ten minutes. Add the beans to the potatoes, and steam for another five minutes. Once cooked, set the potatoes and beans aside to cool. Toast the sunflower or sesame seeds quickly in a dry frying pan until they just begin to brown.

In a large bowl, toss the salad leaves with the Pumpkin Oil Dressing. Mix the vegetables from your minestrone with the leaves. Top with the potatoes, green beans and roasted seeds. Sprinkle with rock or sea salt.

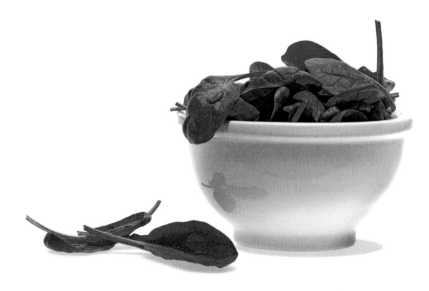

SEARED TUNA, AVOCADO, GINGER, CILANTRO AND LIME

3 oz fresh tuna
1 avocado, peeled and diced
Ginger root, grated
2 tablespoons cilantro,
   chopped

Half a lime
Olive oil
Rock or sea salt
Pepper

Sprinkle enough ginger into a bowl to cover the bottom. Add the chopped cilantro and lime juice. Mix well and season with salt and pepper. Add the avocado to the mix with a dash of olive oil.

Warm a frying pan over high heat and quickly sear the tuna for two minutes on either side, depending on its thickness. You can tell it is done when the color of the fish has changed from dark to light. Plate the tuna and scatter the avocado salad over it.

FILLET OF BEEF WITH BRAISED CELERY AND MASHED SWEET POTATO

1 celery stalk, trimmed
Butter
1 medium sweet potato,
   peeled and chopped

3 oz fillet of beef
Horseradish
Pepper

Place the trimmed celery in a pan and just cover with boiling water. Add a knob of butter and braise slowly for 15 minutes.

In a second pan of boiling water, add the sweet potato and simmer for 15 minutes.

Heat the grill. Once hot, grill the steak. Mash the sweet potato with a little butter and plenty of black pepper. Serve the dish with horseradish.

Ⓥ QUINOA SALAD WITH AVOCADO, TOMATO, PARSLEY AND PINE NUTS

You can vary the grains here and use millet or bulgur wheat, too.

¼ cup quinoa
½ cup water
Handful of parsley,
   finely chopped

1 avocado, peeled, pitted
   and diced
Half a small tomato,
   chopped
Juice of half a grapefruit
10 pine nut kernels

Rinse and drain the quinoa. Add the quinoa and water to a saucepan and, over high heat, bring the water to a boil. Once boiling, place the lid over the saucepan and reduce the heat to low. Let cook for fifteen minutes, then remove the heat. Fluff with a fork and allow to cool. Sprinkle the chopped parsley, avocado and tomato over top the quinoa once it has cooled. Pour the grapefruit juice over the quinoa and toss in the pine nut kernels.

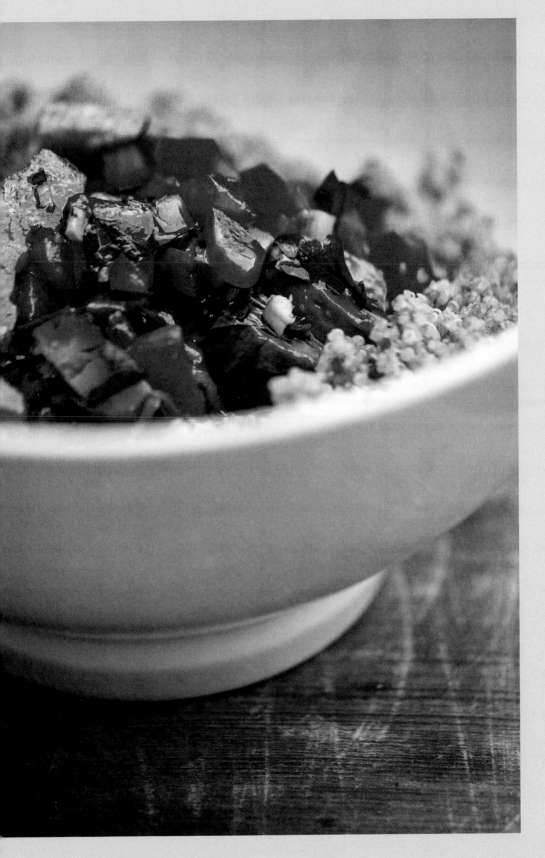

POACHED SALMON, CARROT AND SPINACH MASH AND HEMP SAUCE

1 carrot

2 handfuls of spinach

Nutmeg

Ginger

Bunch of basil

Olive or hemp oil

3 oz salmon fillet

Rock or sea salt

Poach the carrot for ten minutes until soft. Add the spinach for the last two minutes. Drain the carrots and spinach well, and, with a masher or a fork, mash them together with a little vegetable stock. Grate over the nutmeg and a little ginger.

In a blender, mix the basil leaves with a little olive or hemp oil and salt. It should run like a sauce and be vividly green.

Poach the salmon fillet in vegetable stock for two minutes. Serve the salmon on top of the mash and drizzle the green sauce on top.

Ⓥ ROASTED BEET, LIMA BEANS AND CHIVES WITH WALNUT OIL

1 medium beet

¾ cup canned lima beans, rinsed and drained

3 tablespoons chives, cut

Walnut oil

Wrap the beet in silver foil and bake for an hour in a medium oven, about 325°F. You can tell it is cooked when you can slip a knife through easily, like potatoes. Set the beet aside to cool. When cooled, rub off the skin under cold running water. Shake dry and cut into thick slices.

Add the lima beans to the beet and sprinkle the cut chives over the top. Dress with walnut oil.

❤ ASIAN-STYLE STIR-FRY

This is a recipe that we use at the F.X. Mayr & More Health Center because we have access to all these ingredients. You may want to slim it down a little to make at home. Commercial curry spice mixes tend to be alkaline but if you don't like the spiciness you can substitute your Omega Mix (page 140).

Coconut oil

2 inches of ginger root, crushed

1 stalk lemongrass, crushed and diced

2 shiitake mushrooms, chopped

1 small carrot, chopped

10 snow peas

One-quarter of a zucchini, chopped

One-quarter of a leek, chopped

1 cup coconut milk

1 tablespoon curry spice

⅓ cup soaked rice noodles or tofu (or both)

½ cup long green beans, cut

1 bok choy

1 tablespoon cilantro leaves

1 tablespoon Thai basil

Put the coconut oil in a large wok and start to warm. Add the crushed ginger and lemongrass root to the oil to flavor well. Add the vegetables to the wok, mixing well so they pick up the flavors. Add the coconut milk and the curry spice. Stir-fry for three minutes, then add the rice noodles or tofu. Cook for another two minutes. Turn out into a bowl. Quickly boil the green beans and the bok choy together and add to the mix. Finish with the fresh herbs.

♥ ARTICHOKE HEARTS WITH FLAXSEED AND HERB VINAIGRETTE

1 artichoke	1 teaspoon mustard
Flaxseed or olive oil	1 tablespoon fresh
Lemon	herbs, chopped

In a large pan, bring enough water to a boil to cover half the artichoke. Boil for 25 minutes or until the leaves come out easily.

Make up the vinaigrette with flaxseed or olive oil, a squeeze of lemon, a teaspoon of mustard and the chopped herbs.

Eat the leaves first, one at a time. When you get to the base cut out the fine straw core and eat the artichoke heart with a little more herb vinaigrette.

This is a good recipe for eating slowly.

♥ BAKED PEPPER STUFFED WITH BULGUR WHEAT AND NUTS

⅓ cup bulgur wheat	1 tablespoon fresh
3 chestnuts, chopped	parsley, chopped
1 tablespoon pine nuts	Flaxseed or olive oil
	1 red pepper

Set the oven to medium to warm, about 325°F. To make the stuffing, pour boiling water over the bulgur wheat and simmer. Add in the chestnuts and cook for 15 minutes. Strain the bulgur and chestnuts and mix in the pine nuts, chopped herbs and a little oil to moisten.

Cut off the top of the pepper and cut out the seeds. Fill the pepper with the stuffing. Bake the stuffed pepper for 20–25 minutes.

SPICY MEATBALLS WITH TZATZIKI

This alkaline recipe turns the usual (acidic) meatballs and tomato sauce on its head by instead combining meatballs with a classic Greek yogurt sauce that is totally alkaline. All the other ingredients added to the ground beef—the onion, paprika, parsley and bread—are also alkalizing, therefore lessening the acidity of the meat.

1 onion, diced

Coconut oil

3 oz organic ground beef

1 egg

1 slice bread, made into bread crumbs

Paprika

Parsley, chopped

½ cup yogurt

½ cup cucumber slices

3 garlic cloves, crushed

Mint, chopped

Fry the onion in coconut oil until translucent. Meanwhile, mix the meat with the egg, bread crumbs, paprika and chopped parsley (or other herbs). Pour in the cooked onions and roll the mix into small balls. Put them into a frying pan to cook slowly.

To make the tzatziki, mix the yogurt with sliced cucumber, as much crushed garlic as you like and a generous handful of chopped mint. Serve with the meatballs.

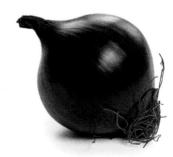

⊘ QUINOA RISOTTO

A quinoa risotto is easier than one made with white rice (and much more alkaline). Use the vegetables left over from your minestrone for this dish to add color.

2 tablespoons curry spice	½ cup quinoa, rinsed
1 small carrot, diced	3 cups water
Half a celery stalk, diced	1 tablespoon cashews
One-quarter of	Lemon zest
a zucchini, diced	3 tablespoons cream
One-quarter of a sweet	or soy cream
potato, diced	Basil leaves, torn

In a frying pan, dry roast the curry spices for a few minutes over high heat until they start to release their oils. Add in the diced vegetables and mix well. Add water and bring to a boil. Simmer for three minutes, then pour in the quinoa. Stir, keeping the mixture moving. Bring back to a boil and simmer for another ten minutes.

While this cooks, toast the cashews in a dry pan until they start to color. When the quinoa is cooked, add in the lemon zest, cream (or soy cream) and cashew nuts. Finish with fresh basil leaves.

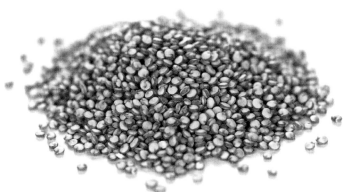

ⓥ GRATIN OF POTATOES, ONIONS AND NUTMEG

1 large potato, sliced
Half an onion, diced
Butter
Organic vegetable stock

Rock or sea salt
Pepper
Nutmeg

Run the sliced potatoes under water to rinse out the starch. Lightly coat a baking tray with butter, and layer the potatoes and onions in it. Half cover with vegetable stock. Season well with salt and pepper. Bake for an hour in a medium to hot oven, about 350°F, until the top is crisp. Serve with a grating of nutmeg.

GRILLED LAMB CHOP WITH FENNEL, CUCUMBER, GRAPEFRUIT AND FIG SALAD

Add grapefruit to the salad if you have some left over from breakfast.

Half a fennel bulb, sliced
Half a cucumber, skinned and sliced lengthwise
Half a grapefruit, segmented

2 figs, opened
2 tablespoons mint, chopped
Parsley oil
1 lamb chop

Turn up the grill to high and leave to heat. Braise the sliced fennel in water for five minutes. Drain and place in a bowl with the cucumber slices, grapefruit segments, opened figs and mint. Put your lamb chop on to grill. Turn halfway through, depending on how rare you like your meat.

DINNER

The earlier you eat dinner, the better, as your body needs time to digest fully before you go to bed. Portion sizes should also be controlled for this same reason. A way to help you adjust your portion sizes for dinner is by using smaller plates. We also recommend that you avoid raw foods after four o'clock in the afternoon because they are harder for your body to digest. A fully cooked vegetable soup is the ideal way to round off your day, but the following recipes provide some delicious, alkaline alternatives. Each recipe typically serves one.

Ⓥ BAKED POTATO WITH ALKALINE MAYONNAISE AND WATERCRESS

A baked potato is such a dependable alkaline food that it deserves to be taken seriously. You can also save the skins and fill with curd and herbs for an emergency lunch.

    1 baking potato
    2 tablespoons Alkaline Mayonnaise (page 169)
    1 tablespoon watercress, chopped
    Rock or sea salt

Bake the potato in the oven for about an hour or until a knife slips in easily. Take it out and set aside to cool slowly until you are ready to eat—it will keep cooking in its own heat. To serve, slice the potato in half and put one tablespoon of Alkaline Mayonnaise on each side and garnish generously with chopped watercress and a sprinkle of rock or sea salt.

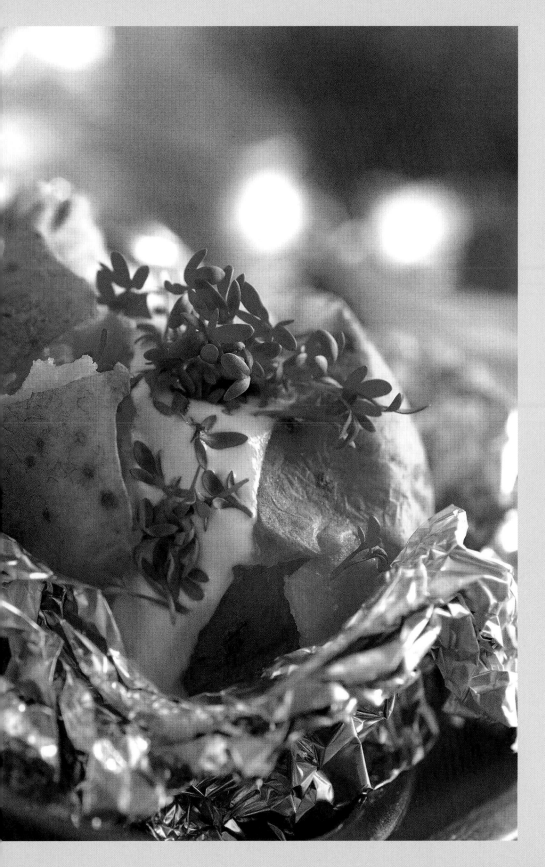

SMOKED MACKEREL AND VEGETABLES WITH PARSLEY OIL

This is a quick, easy supper if you are busy. You can substitute another smoked fish, like smoked trout, if it is easier to find. Horseradish is alkaline but beware—many of the store-bought varieties will be awash with acid ingredients.

3 oz smoked mackerel fillet
Organic vegetable stock
1⅓ cup mixed vegetables
   from your minestrone

2 tablespoon parsley oil
1 tablespoon horseradish,
   shaved

Warm through your mackerel in a little vegetable stock or you can serve it cold.

Skim off the vegetables from your minestrone. Dress with parsley oil and shavings of fresh horseradish.

ⓥ WARM SALAD OF KOHLRABI, BROCCOLI AND CELERIAC IN HERB OIL

This recipe is a bit of a shortcut because the cooking water for the vegetables will give you a stock that you can use for a soup or vegetable stock later on. Just add herbs and spices and simmer for another ten minutes. You can vary the vegetables in this recipe but these go very well together.

Half a small kohlrabi, skinned and chopped
1 large broccoli floret, cut into smaller pieces
Half a small celeriac, skinned and chopped
2 tablespoons Herb Oil (page 168)

In a pot of water, simmer the kohlrabi and celeriac for ten minutes, then add the broccoli florets and cook for another two minutes. Drain and reserve the cooking liquid. Serve the vegetables with herb oil.

❶ ROASTED BEET WITH WALNUT OIL AND CARAWAY SEEDS

1 good-sized beet
Walnut oil
Caraway seeds

Wrap the beet in aluminum foil and bake slowly in the oven. When you can slip a knife easily through the middle, it is cooked—about 45 minutes to an hour, depending on the size. Leave to cool, then peel under cold running water.

Dress with walnut oil and sprinkle with caraway seeds.

❶ BRAISED FENNEL WITH ZUCCHINI

Half a fennel bulb, sliced
Half a zucchini, sliced
1 tablespoon butter

1 tablespoon parsley,
  chopped
Lemon

Slice the fennel lengthways. Place in the bottom of a small pan with just enough water to cover. Bring the water to a boil and allow to cook slowly for ten minutes. Add the zucchini to the mix. Cook for another five minutes. Make sure there is a little water left in the pan. Remove the heat, add the butter and garnish with parsley and a squeeze of lemon.

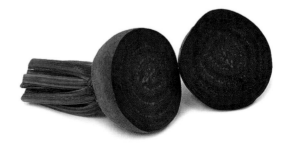

OILS, SAUCES AND DRESSINGS

Oils, sauces and dressings can help bring new flavor dimensions to seemingly plain dishes. Oils, particularly virgin oils, also lend nutritional depth to your food since they are filled with vitamins and essential fatty acids. These oils, sauces and dressings are easy to make and much healthier than most store-bought sauces and dressings.

ⓥ HERB OIL

Herb oils are an exciting way to get the value of the herbs into your diet in different ways. If you use parsley as a base you can add in other herbs for different textures, flavors and nutrients. Mix it up with flaxseed, pumpkin or nut oils for different dimensions. This recipe makes ⅔ cup.

> ¾ cup flat-leaf parsley leaves
> ¾ cup tarragon leaves
> ¾ cup extra-virgin olive oil
> Rock or sea salt

Bring a medium saucepan of water to a boil. Add rock or sea salt to the water.

Blanch the parsley and tarragon (or other fresh herbs) until bright green—just ten seconds or so. Quickly drain and transfer to a bowl of ice water. Drain again and pat with a clean tea towel to remove as much water as possible. Blend in a food processor with the oil until smooth—at least a minute. Strain through a fine sieve or cheese cloth.

You can keep the oil in the refrigerator for up to two weeks.

ⓥ PUMPKIN OIL DRESSING

> 3 parts olive oil
> 1 part pumpkin oil
> 1 part lemon
>
> 2 tablespoons parsley
> or chives, chopped

Mix all of the ingredients together well and serve over a salad or vegetables.

♥ ALKALINE MAYONNAISE

Homemade mayonnaise can be a good vehicle for introducing flaxseed, pumpkin or nut oils into your diet. The yolk of the egg is alkaline. (It is the whites that are acidic.) This recipe makes about 3 cups.

1 egg
1 teaspoon dry mustard
2 cups olive oil

½ cup flaxseed, pumpkin
  or nut oil
Rock or sea salt
Lemon

The eggs should be at room temperature, and it is best if you use older eggs. Separate the egg yolk from the white. Mix the yolk in a bowl with the mustard to form an emulsion. Slowly add the olive oil: stirring the mixture clockwise vigorously, add a small drizzle of olive oil until it is completely incorporated, then add a little more, and a little more. Finally, add the flax or pumpkin oil for flavor.

Season with salt and a squeeze of lemon.

♥ ALMOND PESTO

This recipes works well with the Alkaline Minestrone. This recipe makes about 1 cup.

1 basil plant
2 tablespoon almonds
2 tablespoons Parmesan, grated
Olive, pumpkin, flaxseed or almond oil

Pick the leaves off of the basil plant. Put them in a blender with the almonds and Parmesan. Add two tablespoons of oil and blend. If needed, add more oil to get a thick but manageable paste. Store in a jar and refrigerate; the pesto will keep for a week.

FREQUENTLY
ASKED QUESTIONS

What if I work full time? Can I still take the Alkaline Cure?
Absolutely. This is a very realistic goal. You can prepare your lunches
the day before and warm them up at work. It is important to try to cut
down on stress during the cure. It is also better to be at home for the
cure, so best not to undertake the cure while traveling on business.

If I don't eat meat, wouldn't that mean that I am naturally more alkaline?
Not necessarily. There are many vegetarian foods that are acidic as well
as generally unhealthy. For instance, vegetarian protein sources, such
as cheese and soy, are acid-forming foods. Also, anything alkaline that
isn't chewed sufficiently will turn acidic in your stomach. The key to an
alkaline diet is considering the balance and the quantity of food, and
this applies to vegetarians and meat-eaters alike.

Can I have a glass of wine while I am on the cure?
During the fourteen-day plan it is best to give your system a complete
rest so we advise no alcohol or caffeine. In daily life, a glass of sherry
or wine is no problem—indeed it can even stimulate the digestive
system—but best to avoid anything sparkling, which is automatically
more acidic. Young wines tend to be less acidic than older wines.

Will I be hungry on the cure?
During the first week of the cure, you are likely to have one or two
days when you don't feel great. This is more likely to be sugar cravings
than hunger. Try not to reach for the snack bar but do eat a good
breakfast, keep hydrated and get plenty of rest.

Why don't you have much fruit on the fourteen-day cure?
We like to minimize fiber consumption on the cure in order to be as
gentle on the stomach as possible. Fruit has a lot of sugar as well and
can ferment easily over the course of the fourteen days. Generally
however, fruit is fine in moderation as long as it is ripe. Often the fruit
we eat is not ripe enough and this makes digestion even harder.

What about eating out?

Restaurant menus generally tend to be acidic, although restaurants that use fresher and more expensive ingredients will likely offer some alkaline dishes. Chain restaurants, for the most part, will have acidic menus. If you go out and have a heavily acidic evening just be aware of the imbalance and remember to consume more alkaline foods in your meals for the next few days. Soup is usually a good standby for this.

You recommend eating potatoes. Aren't potatoes fattening?

No—as long they are not deep-fried. They have more potassium than bananas, high vitamin C and B6 content and no calories from fat.

I am on medication—is it safe to follow the Alkaline Cure?

Certainly—it will probably help. Many modern drugs upset the fauna in the stomach and complementing them with an alkaline diet will help you recover quicker. However, you should always check with a medical professional.

Can I be too alkaline?

Yes, but this is a rare condition and not connected to diet. If your pH readings are very alkaline, see a medical professional.

Can I be on an alkaline diet during pregnancy?

The general alkaline diet can be adopted and has been proven to increase fertility. An alkaline environment is beneficial for an unborn child. But it is not advisable to take more extreme parts of the cure such as Epsom salts and baking soda while you are pregnant.

Is the Alkaline Cure suitable for children?

This cure is not advised while children are still growing.

When is the best time to start the cure?

The best time is now.

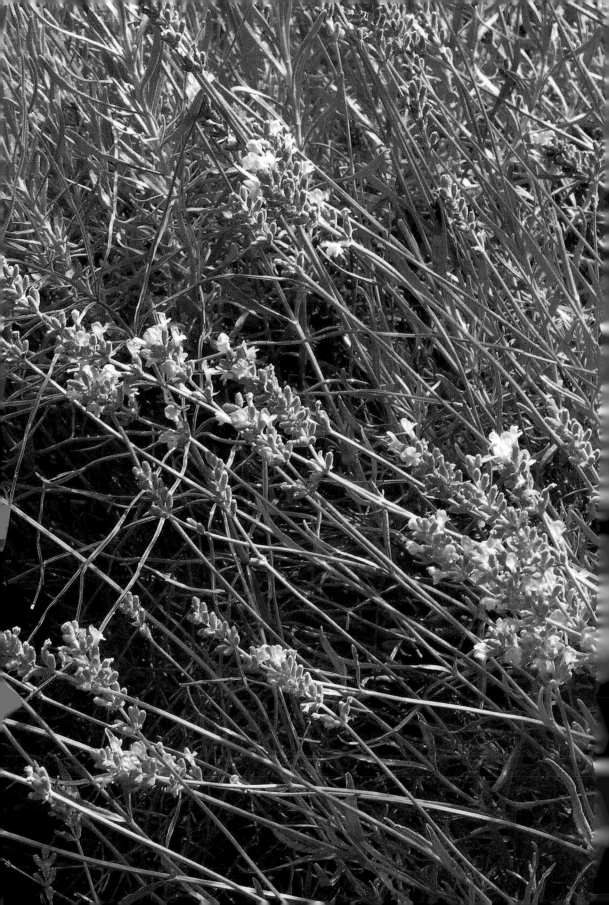

RECIPE FINDER

INDEX

ACKNOWLEDGMENTS

I would like to say thank you to Drew for his unbelievable help, patience, good spirits and wisdom; to Silvia and the team at Elwin Street for the opportunity; to all my patients who have helped me learn; to my teachers Dr. Schulz, Dr. Stossier and Dr. Werner; and, last but not least, to my wife and my children for all of their support and love.

Elwin Street would like to thank everyone at the Original F.X. Mayr & More Health Center for their help in creating this book as well as Susan Levin for her guidance on nutrition. Elwin Street would also like to thank Micro Essential Inc. USA for the supply of these pH strips.

For more information: about the health center, please visit www.mayrandmore. com; about Micro Essential Inc. USA, please visit www.microessentiallab.com. about alkaline recipes, go to www.alkalinecanteen.com.

Resources

Wolfgang Marktl, Bettina Reiter and Cem Ekmekcioglu. 2007. *Säuren-Basen-Schlacken: Pro und Contra—eine wissenschaftliche Diskussion.* Springer Wien New York, Germany.

Dr. F.X. Mayr. 1921. *Fundamente zur Diagnostik de Verdauungskrankheiten* [*Fundamentals of the Diagnosis of Digestive Illnesses*]. Verlag Neues Leben, Austria.

Dr. Erich Rauch. 2008. *Health Through Inner Body Cleansing.* Georg Thieme Verlag, Germany.

Johan van Limburg-Stirum. 2008. *Moderne Säure-Basen-Medezin.* Georg Thieme Verlag, Germany.

Michael Worlitschek. 2008. *Paxis des Säure-Basen Haushalts.* Karl F. Haug Fachbuchverlag, Germany.

Photo Credits

Alessandra Spairani: pp. 10-1, 23, 26-7, 35, 39, 42-3, 51, 62-3, 65, 73, 79, 91, 94-5, 99, 117, 135, 136-7, 143, 157; Dreamstime: pp. 89, 103, 140, 167; Drew Smith: pp. 18, 40, 58, 172; Getty: pp. 55, 74, 147, 165; iStock: pp. 7, 13, 30, 45, 49, 84, 101, 105, 107, 108, 111, 112, 115, 119, 120, 123, 125, 126, 128, 131, 133, 154, 161, 162; The Original F.X. Mayr & More Health Center: pp. 3, 8